Surgery and the Geriatric Patient

Editors

FRED A. LUCHETTE
ROBERT D. BARRACO

CLINICS IN GERIATRIC MEDICINE

www.geriatric.theclinics.com

February 2019 • Volume 35 • Number 1

ELSEVIER

1600 John F. Kennedy Boulevard • Suite 1800 • Philadelphia, Pennsylvania, 19103-2899

http://www.theclinics.com

CLINICS IN GERIATRIC MEDICINE Volume 35, Number 1
February 2019 ISSN 0749–0690, ISBN-13: 978-0-323-65449-4

Editor: Jessica McCool
Developmental Editor: Laura Fisher

Clinics in Geriatric Medicine (ISSN 0749-0690) is published quarterly by Elsevier Inc., 360 Park Avenue South, New York, NY 10010-1710. Months of issue are February, May, August, and November. Business and Editorial Offices: 1600 John F. Kennedy Blvd., Suite 1800, Philadelphia, PA 191023-2899. Periodicals postage paid at New York, NY, and additional mailing offices. Subscription prices are $286.00 per year (US individuals), $632.00 per year (US institutions), $100.00 per year (US student/resident), $320.00 per year (Canadian individuals), $801.00 per year (Canadian institutions), $195.00 per year (Canadian student/resident), $402.00 per year (international individuals), $801.00 per year (international institutions), and $195.00 per year (international student/resident). Foreign air speed delivery is included in all *Clinics* subscription prices. All prices are subject to change without notice. POSTMASTER: Send address changes to *Clinics in Geriatric Medicine*, Elsevier Health Sciences Division, Subscription Customer Service, 3251 Riverport Lane, Maryland Heights, MO 63043. **Telephone: 1-800-654-2452 (U.S. and Canada); 314-447-8871 (outside U.S. and Canada). Fax: 314-447-8029.** E-mail: journalscustomerservice-usa@elsevier.com **(for print support)** or journalsonlinesupport-usa@elsevier.com **(for online support).**

Reprints. For copies of 100 or more, of articles in this publication, please contact the Commercial Reprints Department, Elsevier Inc., 360 Park Avenue South, New York, New York 10010-1710. Tel.: 212-633-3874; Fax: 212-633-3820, E-mail: reprints@elsevier.com.

Clinics in Geriatric Medicine is covered in *MEDLINE/PubMed (Index Medicus), EMBASE/Excerpta Medica, Current Contents/Clinical Medicine (CC/CM),* and the *Cumulative Index to Nursing & Allied Health Literature.*

Contributors

EDITORS

FRED A. LUCHETTE, MD, MSc
Vice Chair of VA Affairs, Professor of Surgery, Department of Surgery, Stritch School of Medicine, Loyola University Chicago, Chief of Surgical Services, Edward Hines Jr. VA Medical Center, Maywood, Illinois

ROBERT D. BARRACO, MD, MPH
Chief Academic Officer, Lehigh Valley Health Network, Associate Dean for Educational Affairs, Professor of Surgery, Department of Surgery, University of South Florida Morsani College of Medicine, Lehigh Valley Campus, Allentown, Pennsylvania

AUTHORS

JESSICA H. BALLOU, MD, MPH
Surgical Resident, Department of Surgery, Oregon Health & Science University, Portland, Oregon

DEBORAH J. BOLDING, PhD
Occupational Therapist, Trauma Service, Stanford Health Care, Assistant Professor, San Jose State University, San Jose, California

KAREN J. BRASEL, MD, MPH, FACS
Professor, Department of Surgery, Oregon Health & Science University, Portland, Oregon

STEVEN E. BROOKS, MD, FACS
Associate Professor of Surgery and Chief, Division of Trauma and Surgical Critical Care, Department of Surgery, Texas Tech University Health Sciences Center, Lubbock, Texas

SIGRID K. BURRUSS, MD, FACS
Assistant Professor of Surgery, Director of Trauma Prevention and Outreach, Division of Acute Care Surgery, Loma Linda University Medical Center, Loma Linda, California

ELLEN CORMAN, MRA
Manager, Injury Prevention and Community Engagement, Trauma Service, Stanford Health Care/Stanford Medicine, Stanford, California

MARIE CRANDALL, MD, MPH, FACS
Professor and Associate Chair for Research, Department of Surgery, University of Florida College of Medicine Jacksonville, Jacksonville, Florida

MOUSTAPHA DIMACHK, MD
Resident, Department of Surgery, University of Florida College of Medicine Jacksonville, Jacksonville, Florida

JAMES K. DZANDU, PhD
HonorHealth John C. Lincoln Hospital, Phoenix, Arizona

JOHN T. GORCZYCA, MD
Dr. C. McCollister Evarts Professor in Orthopaedics, Department of Orthopaedics, University of Rochester Medical Center, Rochester, New York

WENDY R. GREENE, MD, FACS, FCCM
Emory University School of Medicine, Atlanta, Georgia

ALEXANDER S. GREENSTEIN, MD
Orthopaedic Surgery Resident, Department of Orthopaedics, University of Rochester Medical Center, Rochester, New York

SHAILVI GUPTA, MD, MPH
Surgical Critical Care Fellow, Shock Trauma Center, University of Maryland School of Medicine, Baltimore, Maryland

PEGGE M. HALANDRAS, MD
Associate Professor, Department of Vascular Surgery and Endovascular Surgery, Stritch School of Medicine, Loyola University Chicago, Maywood, Illinois

MOHAMMAD HAMIDI, MD
Research Fellow, Department of Surgery, Division of Trauma, Critical Care and Emergency Surgery, The University of Arizona, Tucson, Arizona

MICHAEL E. JOHNSTON II, MD
Department of Surgery, University of Cincinnati College of Medicine, Cincinnati, Ohio

BELLAL JOSEPH, MD, FACS
Professor, Department of Surgery, Division of Trauma, Critical Care and Emergency Surgery, The University of Arizona, Tucson, Arizona

ROSEMARY KOZAR, MD, PhD
Professor of Surgery, Shock Trauma Center, University of Maryland School of Medicine, Baltimore, Maryland

ALICIA J. MANGRAM, MD, FACS
Valley Surgical Clinics and Acute Care Surgical Specialists, HonorHealth John C. Lincoln Hospital, Phoenix, Arizona

CATHY A. MAXWELL, PhD, RN
Assistant Professor, Vanderbilt University School of Nursing, Nashville, Tennessee

RICHARD S. MILLER, MD, FACS
Chief, Division of Trauma and Surgical Critical Care, Vanderbilt University Medical Center, Nashville, Tennessee

KAUSHIK MUKHERJEE, MD, MSCI, FACS
Assistant Professor of Surgery, Associate Trauma Medical Director, Division of Acute Care Surgery, Loma Linda University Medical Center, Loma Linda, California

MAYUR B. PATEL, MD, MPH
Assistant Professor of Surgery, Division of Trauma and Surgical Critical Care, Vanderbilt University Medical Center, Nashville, Tennessee

SAMEER H. PATEL, MD
Division of Surgical Oncology, Assistant Professor, Department of Surgery, University of Cincinnati College of Medicine, Cincinnati, Ohio

JUSTIN A. PERRY, MSW
Department of Care Management, University of Maryland Medical Center, Baltimore, Maryland

RANDI SMITH, MD
Emory University School of Medicine, Grady Hospital, Atlanta, Georgia

LUIS C. SUAREZ-RODRIGUEZ, MD
Clinical Fellow, Division of Trauma and Surgical Critical Care, Vanderbilt University Medical Center, Nashville, Tennessee

JOSEPH F. SUCHER, MD, FACS
Valley Surgical Clinics and Acute Care Surgical Specialists, HonorHealth Deer Valley Hospital, Phoenix, Arizona

JEFFREY J. SUSSMAN, MD
Professor, Department of Surgery, University of Cincinnati College of Medicine, Cincinnati, Ohio

ASTRID BOTTY VAN DEN BRUELE, MD
Resident, Department of Surgery, University of Florida College of Medicine Jacksonville, Jacksonville, Florida

Contents

pain and other symptoms to maintain the highest quality of life for the longest period of time, but surgical patients are less likely to be referred to palliative care than patients with chronic medical conditions. Meeting the palliative care needs of elderly surgical patients requires early recognition, advance care planning, and multidisciplinary interventions that align patient goals with possible outcomes.

Elderly patients are at increased risk for morbidity and mortality after injury or surgery in both the inpatient and postdischarge settings. The importance of discharge destination after the index hospitalization is increasingly recognized as a determinant of long-term survival, with discharge to a post–acute care facility portending a worse prognosis. Efforts to minimize discharge to post–acute care facilities should include early discharge planning. Communication among a multidisciplinary care team sets the groundwork for effective discharge planning and transitions of care. The elderly face several systematic, psychosocial, functional, and financial barriers that pose significant challenges to successful transitions of care.

Geriatric medicine is a growing field filled with complicated patients who are susceptible to developing cancer. Surgical oncology is expanding while adapting to the increasing elderly population and creating novel treatment regimens for this group of patients. This article reviews surgical oncology in elderly patients and addresses surgical optimization, management of several cancer subtypes, surgical advances in minimally invasive surgery, and ethical considerations.

As more patients live longer, it is probable that an increasing number of geriatric patients will require surgery. An organized, systematic, coordinated, multidisciplinary approach to the perioperative management of these patients will result in fewer complications, improved outcomes, and reduced cost of care. Details are herein provided on the preoperative diagnostic evaluation and assessment as well as perioperative care provided to optimize outcomes. The diagnosis, workup, and treatment of osteoporosis and fragility fractures are presented. The article concludes with a review of the care of the geriatric orthopedic patient in the posthospital time period.

As the population ages, surgical decision-making in vascular surgery has become more complex. Older patients may not have been offered vascular surgical intervention in the past because of prohibitive physiologic demands and poor health. Patients now have more aggressive management of vascular risk factors with medications, such as statin therapy, and less invasive endovascular or hybrid treatment options. Outcomes in elderly patients may not be comparable with younger patients for entities such as aortic aneurysm repair, carotid endarterectomy, or lower extremity revascularization. Despite this, desirable outcomes can be successfully achieved and should be offered to carefully selected elderly individuals.

illness, loss of functional status, isolation, and family, financial, and social factors. Access to firearms is another significant risk factor, because elderly patients are more likely to use firearms in suicide attempts; interventions to reduce firearms mortality may save lives. Tackling the difficult problem of suicide in the elderly may require a multidisciplinary, community-based series of interventions.

CLINICS IN GERIATRIC MEDICINE

FORTHCOMING ISSUES

May 2019
Falls Prevention
Steven C. Castle, *Editor*

August 2019
Anemia in Older Adults
William B. Ershler, *Editor*

November 2019
Cardiac Rehabilitation
Daniel E. Forman, *Editor*

RECENT ISSUES

November 2018
Alzheimer Disease and Other Dementias
John E. Morley, *Editor*

August 2018
Care for the Older Adult in the Emergency Department
Michael L. Malone and Kevin Biese, *Editors*

May 2018
Geriatric Otolaryngology
Karen M. Kost, *Editor*

SERIES OF RELATED INTEREST

Surgical Clinics
Medical Clinics
Primary Care: Clinics in Office Practice

Preface

Nuances of Surgical Care for the Elderly

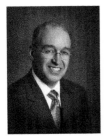 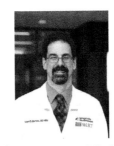

Fred A. Luchette, MD, MSc   Robert D. Barraco, MD, MPH
Editors

Unprecedented population growth, complex medical problems, and widespread use of anticoagulants: the perfect storm for the Silver Tsunami. Those aged 65 and over will number 98.2 million in the United States in the year 2060, with 19.7 million aged 85 and over.[1] Arthritis, heart disease, cancer, pulmonary disease, and Alzheimer round out the top five health concerns in the elderly per the Centers for Disease Control and Prevention. However, the unspoken epidemic is that of frailty, with 44% of the elderly prefrail and 10% frail.[2] Anticoagulants have reduced stroke rates and now come in forms that need no laboratory testing. However, many are without antidotes, and combined with a rate of falls at 25%, contribute to poor outcomes.

This issue of *Clinics in Geriatric Medicine* focuses on the surgical care of this vulnerable population, giving caregivers the information they need to improve care. We begin with the changing epidemiology of Baby Boomers to Elder Explosion. Frailty and its effect on prognostication are important for establishing goals of care for the team. Geriatric Consultation and Team-Based Care along with Palliative Care are being introduced into practice at many centers. Transitions of care are so important for this population to be sure that care implemented in the hospital carries over to the outpatient setting or skilled nursing facility.

The elderly pose many unique problems for the care teams in cancer care, orthopedics, and vascular surgery. Last, the authors address major issues in injury prevention for the elderly. Elder abuse is a pervasive problem that is underreported and not easily identified. Falls remain the most common cause of admission in the elderly, expected to cost almost $70 billion in 2020, with $52 billion of that to Medicare.[3] One of the most difficult issues for practitioners is when to ask the patient to turn over the keys to the car and thus reduce their independence. The rate of suicide in the elderly is second only to younger adults aged 45 to 64 years.[4]

Clin Geriatr Med 35 (2019) xiii–xiv
https://doi.org/10.1016/j.cger.2018.10.001
0749-0690/19/© 2018 Published by Elsevier Inc.

geriatric.theclinics.com

We hope that addressing these topics will help providers understand the unique nuances required when caring for surgical patients or the injured elder. Understanding these patient needs should improve patient outcomes.

Fred A. Luchette, MD, MSc
Department of Surgery
Stritch School of Medicine
Loyola University of Chicago
Edward Hines Jr VA Medical Center
2160 South First Avenue
Maywood, IL 60153, USA

Robert D. Barraco, MD, MPH
Lehigh Valley Health Network
Department of Surgery
University of South Florida
Morsani College of Medicine
Lehigh Valley Campus
Department of Education
1247 South Cedar Crest Boulevard
Suite 202
Allentown, PA 18103, USA

E-mail addresses:
fluchet@lumc.edu (F.A. Luchette)
Robert_D.Barraco@lvhn.org (R.D. Barraco)

REFERENCES

1. United States Census Bureau. Facts for features: older Americans month: May 2017. Available at: https://www.census.gov/newsroom/facts-for-features/2017/cb17-ff08.html. Accessed April 20, 2018.
2. Collard RM, Boter H, Schoevers RA, et al. Prevalence of frailty in community-dwelling older persons: a systematic review. J Am Geriatr Soc 2012;60(8):1487–92.
3. National Council on Aging. Issue brief: funding for elder falls prevention. Available at: https://www.ncoa.org/wp-content/uploads/Falls-Funding-Issue-Brief-8-15.pdf. Accessed May 1, 2018.
4. American Foundation for Suicide Prevention. Suicide statistics. Available at: https://afsp.org/about-suicide/suicide-statistics/. Accessed April 20, 2018.

Changing Epidemiology of the American Population

Mohammad Hamidi, MD, Bellal Joseph, MD*

KEYWORDS

- Changing epidemiology • Geriatrics • Geriatric surgery • Cost of caring
- Demographics

KEY POINTS

- Improved life expectancy and enhanced health care system services have led to pronounced epidemiologic changes among the US geriatric population.
- Patient's demographics, injury characteristics, and conditions that require surgical intervention among the growing geriatric population are progressively changing.
- The elderly population receive more medical attention than any other US demographic and have the highest health care spending compared with other age groups in the United States.

INTRODUCTION

The multifaceted, changing epidemiology of geriatric patients has important social, medical, and ethical ramifications that will continue to evolve over the next few decades. Similarly, geriatric surgical care has unique challenges, because older patients have physiologic and social characteristics distinct from their younger counterparts.[1] Consequently, surgeons need to pay special attention to how dynamic changes in this population subset can dramatically affect the perioperative setting and outcomes associated with surgical management. Epidemiology is an arm of medical studies that deals specifically with the incidence, distribution, possible control, and prevention of diseases, and many other factors related to health issues. This article discusses, in brief, the increasing number of older citizens in the US population, transformations in the epidemiology and demographics of geriatric patients, as well as changes in mechanism of injury in this subgroup. We also assess changes in 5 major surgical subspecialties for geriatric patients.

Disclosure Statement: The authors have nothing to disclose.
Department of Surgery, Division of Trauma, Critical Care and Emergency Surgery, The University of Arizona, 1501 North Campbell Avenue, Room 5411, PO Box 245063, Tucson, AZ 85724, USA
* Corresponding author.
E-mail address: bjoseph@surgery.arizona.edu

The Aging Population of the United States

A population's age composition can change through a dynamic process of birth, death, and migration. Changes in the number of newborns have the most impact on the overall age groups. Even though fertility rates have decreased significantly in most regions of the globe, the world population is steadily and rapidly growing as life expectancy has improved owing to advanced health care services. Between 2014 and 2060, according to the US Census Bureau, the total US population is expected to increase from 319 million to 417 million, reaching 400 million by 2051.[2] However, the US population is expected to grow more slowly in future decades than it has in the recent past.

In 2012, the total world population aged 65 and over reached approximately 562 million, constituting 8% of Earth's human population at the time (7 billion).[3] Three years later, in 2015, this segment increased by 55 million (0.5% increase) and became 8.5% of the world's population.[3]

In the 1860s, 50% of the US population was under the age of 20, and most of the population was not expected to live to age 65.[4] As fertility declined and the chances of survival improved, along with enhanced health care services, the American population became progressively older. Some of the most significant future demographic changes expected to take place in the United States include that 20% of the population will be older than 65 years by 2030, more than 50% will belong to a minority group (ie, any group other than non-Hispanic white) by 2044, and nearly 20% will be foreign born by 2060.[2]

Changing Demographics in the Geriatrics

Sex ratio

Sex ratio is defined as the number of males for every 100 females. It is a measure of gender composition in a population. According to the 2010 US Census Report, the ratio of elderly females to males increases with increasing age; this change is most pronounced for those 85 years and older (**Fig. 1**). It is projected that the 1980s ratio of 44

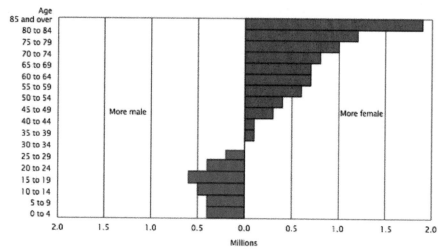

Fig. 1. Difference between male and female populations by age: 2010. (*From* West LA, Cole S, Goodkind D, et al. 65 + in the United States: 2010. Available at: https://www.census.gov/content/dam/Census/library/publications/2014/demo/p23-212.pdf. Accessed March 20, 2018.)

males to 100 females will decrease to 36 males per 100 females by 2020. Thus, it is expected that the vast majority of health problems will occur more commonly in females than males.[5]

Race

The changing racial makeup of the older population is a dynamic process. In 2010, according to the US Census Bureau,[6] almost 85% of the older population identified their race as white, 8.5% Black, 3.4% Asian, and 6.9% Hispanic. The non-Hispanic white race is expected to make up the majority of the older population until 2050. Nonetheless, the elderly population aged 65 and older is expected to become more racially and ethnically diverse.[6] The changing racial distribution of the elderly population between 2000 and 2010 is shown in **Table 1**.

Geographic distribution

Similar to sex ratio and race, the geographic distribution of the US population is also changing over time. In the period between 1990 and 2000, the largest number of elderly people were concentrated in the western and southern regions.[7] In 2000, Florida, Pennsylvania, and West Virginia had the highest number of elderly citizens aged 65 and older.[7] By 2010, 11 states had more than 1 million elderly residents; California had the highest number of elderly, followed by Florida and New York.[6] The geographic distribution of the elderly (aged ≥65 years) by state is demonstrated in **Fig. 2**. As can be seen, multiple geographic disparities of elderly distribution do exist in America. These differences in state and regional density of elderly citizens delineate differential use of health care services.

Acute versus chronic illness

In contrast with the past, the leading cause of death among today's geriatric population is shifting from acute to chronic illnesses. Chronic medical conditions are defined as conditions that last a year or more. These conditions limit the activities of daily living and require continuous and close medical attention, especially in the geriatric population.[8] This paradigmatic shift constitutes a major challenge and burden for the health care system. As of 2012, almost 50% of the adults in America had 1 or more chronic medical conditions.[9] Among the elderly, current statistics demonstrate that 3 of 4 persons aged 65 and older suffer from some kind of chronic medical illness.[10] Providing care for elderly patients with multiple chronic medical conditions accounts for more than two-thirds of the total health care expenditure in the United States, and it has led to an increase of about 90% in Medicare spending.[11,12] Hence, there is a continuous and pressing need for more high-quality, research-based care for this subgroup to improve patient outcomes and minimize associated financial burdens.

Table 1 Distribution of elderly by race		
Race	2000 (%)	2010 (%)
White	86.9	84.8
Black	8.1	8.5
Asian	2.3	3.4
Hispanics	5.0	6.9

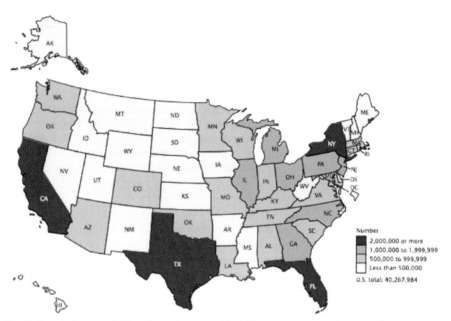

Fig. 2. Population aged 65 and over by state: 2010. (*From* West LA, Cole S, Goodkind D, et al. 65 + in the United States: 2010. Available at: https://www.census.gov/content/dam/Census/library/publications/2014/demo/p23-212.pdf. Accessed March 20, 2018; and U.S. Census Bureau, 2010a; 2010 Census.)

The Cost of Caring for Geriatric Patients

As the elderly US population grows, the demand for health care services and the cost of health care use are expected to continue increasing. Hospital admissions among the geriatric population has reached 40% of the total hospitalized adults, as reported in 2008.[13] In 2015, there was an incremental increase of 0.2% (from 17.7% to 17.9%) in the overall share of the gross domestic product related to health care expenditures.[14] Recently, according to the Centers for Medicare and Medicaid, government health care spending increased 4.3%, totaling $3.3 trillion or approximately $10,348 per citizen.[14]

As per the "Medical Spending of the U.S. Elderly" report, economists Nardi and colleagues[15] made the following findings:

- The US government covers around 65% of the total medical expenditure of the elderly population.
- Medical expenditure for elderly aged 79 to 90 is more than double of the national average, with the highest increase in spending on nursing homes.
- The average medical expenditure in the last year of life is $59,100, of which Medicare covers approximately 71% of the cost, whereas Medicaid covers only 10%.

Among the elderly, falls are the leading cause of fatal and nonfatal injuries.[16] With the increasing number of elderly, there will be a concomitant increase in both the incidence of fall injuries and the cost of treatment, which will further stress the budget for care, including hospitalizations and rehabilitative services.[17] In 2015, it was estimated that the total cost of deaths from fall-related injuries was nearly $637.2 million (56% was spent on females and 44% on males).[18] Regarding nonfatal falls in the same year, the cost was estimated to be $31.3 billion (71% was spent on females and

29% on males).[18] Comparing these costs with those from 10 years earlier, the estimated direct medical costs for nonfatal falls was $19 billion.[19] In other words, the cost of nonfatal falls increased by almost 1.5 fold in 10 years when compared with the cost in 2005.

Changing Injury Epidemiology in the Geriatric Population

Injury in the geriatric population represents an important and increasing public health concern. The epidemiology of injuries in this population is dissimilar to that of younger people. Geriatric patients have their own unique set of interrelated host, agent, and environmental factors that often put them at an increased risk of adverse outcomes from minor injuries. Rhee and colleagues[20] analyzed mortality data over an 11-year period and found that trauma deaths increased by 22.8% from 2000. The most significant increase was noticed in people aged between 45 and 64 years in 2010. Additionally, the highest percent change was in the 54-year-old group. A better understanding of the unique epidemiology of geriatric injuries will lead to improved prevention efforts as well as more effective clinical care paradigms, which will minimize death and disability among the elderly.

In the United States, for both males and females and across all races, unintentional injury is the fifth leading cause of death over all age groups.[21] In 2009, more than 44,000 geriatric people died from injuries, which is equivalent to 120 deaths each day or 1 person every 12 minutes.[22] Geriatric patients are also at an increased risk for fatal injuries, a risk that increases with each year of age. In 2010, the rate of death owing to injury in 65 to 74-year-olds was 60 in 100,000 people, for 75 to 84-year-olds it was 124.7 in 100,000, and for those older than 85 years it was 350 in 100,000. These prevalences compare with a rate of 58 in 100,000 for the general population.[23] Injuries in the elderly are associated with high rates of morbidity that impact personal, family, and societal factors resulting in decreased quality of life and increased cost of immediate and long-term medical care.

Falls

Falls are common in the elderly. They result in a tremendous amount of morbidity, mortality, and consumption of health care services, including admission to assisted living facilities (eg, skilled nursing facilities). In America, approximately 75% of deaths from falls are in the population aged 65 and older. This finding is indicative of a primarily geriatric syndrome. About 40% of the geriatric citizens who live at home are expected to experience at least 1 fall from standing each year. Furthermore, 1 in 40 will be admitted to a hospital for care. Of those requiring admission, only 50% will be alive 1 year later. Repeated falls are a common reason for admission to a skilled nursing facility.[24] The National Health Interview Survey reports that falls account for around 18% of restricted activity days in the geriatric population. Additionally, fall-related injuries account for about 6% of all medical expenditures for geriatric patients. Surprisingly, the US Public Health Service has estimated that potentially two-thirds of fatalities owing to falls are preventable.

Motor vehicle collision

In 2008, there were 30 million licensed drivers aged 65 and older. In the same year, more than 5500 of these drivers died and an additional 180,000 were injured in a motor vehicle collision. As drivers age, the risk of a fatal collision increases in a nonlinear fashion; per mile traveled, it begins to increase at age 75 years and increases sharply after the age of 80.[25] For the oldest drivers, the deadly crash rate increases from around 2 per 100 million miles traveled to more than 12 per 100 million miles traveled.[26] In 2015, there were 40 million licensed drivers aged 65 and older.[27] Thus, there have been 10 million new elderly drivers added to the roadways since 2008. It is projected that there will be an increase in the number of elderly drivers who die or sustain injuries owing to motor vehicle collisions.

Assault and domestic abuse

Geriatric abuse is a growing problem in both social and public health domains. The overall lifetime prevalence of geriatric abuse ranges from 2% to 3%.[28] According to Adult Protective Services, almost one-half of a million cases of mistreatment were reported in 2004,[29] which constitutes about a 20% increase from 2000.[30] Unfortunately, after Adult Protective Services intervention, 14% to 42% of geriatric patients continue to be mistreated.[31] Risk factors associated with geriatric abuse are multifactorial. They include being female, caregivers suffering from stress and a lack of proper coping skills, neurocognitive impairment disorders, and comorbidities like dementia and depression.[32]

Penetrating injuries

The elderly tend to have higher complication and mortality rates after experiencing physical trauma compared with younger patients. Morris and colleagues[33] found a cutoff at the age of 40 years when mortality rates start to increase after injury. Penetrating injuries in the elderly account for a significant number of deaths. A study that analyzed 100,000 gunshot wounds using the National Trauma Databank found that the overall mortality rate in the geriatric population was 40%.[34] Most cases of penetrating wounds in the elderly are self-inflicted related to chronic disease(s) and/or mental illnesses (eg, depression). **Table 2** summarizes the incidence of self-inflicted gunshot wounds in different age groups.[34] According to the American Association of Suicidology, firearms are the most common method (72.1%) used to commit suicide among the elderly. Furthermore, the overall incidence of suicide in the elderly is 14 in 100,00 compared with 11 in 100,000 in the general population.[35]

Geriatric Surgery in the United States

It is well-known that the elderly population is rapidly increasing in America. Over the past 20 years, the proportion of elderly patients requiring surgery has outpaced this growth rate. Currently, more than 50% of the surgeries in the United States are performed on elderly patients.[36] In this section, we will briefly review the changing epidemiology of surgery for elderly patients undergoing emergency surgery, bariatric surgery, cardiothoracic surgery, orthopedic surgery, and neurosurgery.

Emergency general surgery

As the US population gets older, the incidence of emergency general surgery among the elderly is increasing. In this subsection, we demonstrate the changing

Table 2	
Self-inflected gunshot wounds in different age groups	
Age Group (y)	Incidence (%)
55–64	29.2
65–74	46.2
≥75	51.5

epidemiology of 2 common emergency general surgery procedures, namely, acute appendicitis and acute cholecystitis.

Acute appendicitis In the elderly, appendicitis constitutes 14% of all abdominal emergencies. However, 80% of the patients are younger than 50 years.[37] In the group older than 50 years, 1 in 35 females and 1 in 50 males will eventually develop appendicitis during their lifetime.[38] Overall, between 1993 and 2008, the incidence of acute appendicitis increased from 7.62 in 10,000 people to 9.38 in 10,000 people. Concurrently, there was an increase of 6.3% in those 30 to 69 years of age.[39] During the same period, the rates of acute appendicitis increased in Hispanics, Native Americans, and Asians, whereas the frequencies among whites and blacks were decreasing.[39] The changing demographic makeup of the United States might be the reason for these changes.

Acute cholecystitis Biliary tract disorders are among the top reasons for surgery and hospital admission in elderly patients. For patients in their 70s, the incidence of biliary disease is 50% for females and 16% for males.[40] Thus, surgery for symptomatic cholelithiasis is more common in the elderly because the incidence of gallstones increases with age (the incidence is around 13%–50% in patients above the age of 70 and 38%–50% in those above the age of 80).[41] Improvements in technical skills and advances in technology have led to more favorable outcomes with laparoscopic cholecystectomy. For example, Bingener and colleagues[40] have demonstrated improvement in outcomes in elderly patients undergoing laparoscopic cholecystectomy over a 10-year period (1991–2001). The conversion rate has dropped from 17% to 7%. Similarly, the average hospital duration of stay has decreased from 10.2 days to 4.6 days. The improvement in the conversion rate was mainly attributed to the lower rate of complications during the laparoscopic procedure, better ability to identify diverse anatomy, and enhanced laparoscopic manipulation skills of the surgeons, which is accompanied by increased experience with laparoscopic procedures.

Bariatric surgery
Obesity is a known cause of decreased quality of life and life expectancy.[42] Bariatric procedures include sleeve gastrectomy and Roux-en-Y gastric bypass, among others. Collectively, they are considered the most effective treatments for morbid obesity.[43] There is a trend toward increased numbers of sleeve gastrectomies and fewer bypass procedures being performed.[44] As the US population ages, the number of morbidly obese elderly patients requiring bariatric surgery is projected to increase. In 1991, almost 15% of the elderly population aged 60 to 69 and 11.4% of those over the age of 70 were obese.[45] In 2000, the prevalence of obesity increased by 56% and by 36% in these 2 groups, respectively.[46] The low incidence of obesity in those greater than 80 years of age could be attributed to the survival advantage for the nonobese.[47] This increment in the obesity prevalence among elderly has led to an expansion in the number of bariatric surgeries performed and covered by Medicare.[48]

Cardiothoracic surgery
The epidemiology of patients undergoing cardiothoracic surgical procedures is also changing. According to The National Hospital Discharge Survey, between 1996 and 2006, the number of coronary artery bypass grafting procedures decreased by 31%. In contrast, the number of operations for valvular disease increased by 26%. The incidence of these procedures is different in elderly age groups. The population-based incidence rate for coronary artery bypass grafting has decreased by 38% from 1996 to 2006. Decreases were most pronounced in the age groups with the highest frequency of operations (60–79 years old). However, coronary artery

bypass grafting incidence rates in those aged 80 and older were unchanged. In contrast, the rate of valve procedures and pneumonectomies remained constant over the same period. Over the next few decades, as the US population continues to age, the field of cardiothoracic surgery will experience a significant increase in its patient base despite a continual decrease in the incidence rates of heart and lung diseases.[49]

Orthopedic surgery

The aging global population is expected to cause a substantial increase in the demand for orthopedic surgery. Particular orthopedic procedures that are more prevalent in the elderly include joint replacement, spine procedures, and foot and ankle operations. Cram and colleagues[50] analyzed trends and outcomes for primary and revisional knee replacement in patients aged 65 and older between 1991 and 2010. They found that the annual volume of primary knee replacement increased by 161%, and by 106% for revision of a prior replacement. Despite these increases, there was a decrease in the hospital duration of stay for both procedures. Another study by Yoshihara and colleagues[51] found that there is an overall increase in the rates of elective major orthopedic operations in patients aged 80 years and above in the United States. This increase was accompanied by a decrease in the rate of in-hospital mortality and stable rates of in-hospital complications. These outcomes indicate an enhancement in the health care services.

Spinal and central nervous system procedures

Aging is accompanied by degenerative changes in the spine, including herniation of intervertebral discs, osteophyte formation, and fractures.[52] These degenerative changes are associated with an increased demand for surgical intervention, especially among patients over the age of 65.[53] Ciol and colleagues[54] studied the epidemiology of surgery for spinal stenosis in patients aged 65 and older. They concluded that, from 1979 to 1992, the rate of operations for spinal stenosis increased 8-fold. Furthermore, in the period between 1988 and 2001, the rate of lumbar fusion procedures increased by 230%.[55] Recently, rates of decompression surgery and simple fusions decreased from 2002 to 2007; however, rates of complex fusion surgeries increased 15-fold.[56]

The incidence of chronic subdural hematoma (SDH) is increasing as Americans live longer, However, the neurologic outcomes in the elderly are relatively poor and usually result in serious disability.[57] The 1-year mortality rate can be as high as 32% among elderly patients who undergo simple drainage for SDH.[58] Balser and colleagues[59] predicted that by 2030, the incidence of chronic SDH will reach 17.6 cases per 100,000 in the general US population. If correct, in 2030 the most commonly performed neurosurgical procedure may be drainage of SDH.

SUMMARY

- The US population is aging, in parallel with improved life expectancy and enhanced health care system services.
- The demographics of the geriatric population are dynamic variables, and they are projected to be even more diverse in the near future.
- As the US population becomes older, the demand for health care services will continue to increase, and the total medical expenditure and financial burden will increase.
- Injury patterns and characteristics are also continuously changing among the elderly. A comprehensive understanding of these patterns is crucial to aid in the development of effective prevention strategies.

- The proportion of elderly patients requiring specialty surgery in the United States is outpacing the continuous growth of the population.

REFERENCES

1. Evers BM, Townsend CM Jr, Thompson JC. Organ physiology of aging. Surg Clin North Am 1994;74(1):23–39.
2. Colby SL, Ortman JM. Projections of the size and composition of the US population: 2014 to 2060, 9. Washington, DC: US Census Bureau; 2015.
3. National Research Council, Committee on Population, Committee on National Statistics. Preparing for an aging world: the case for cross-national research. Washington, DC: National Academies Press; 2001.
4. Hobbs F, Damon BL. Sixty-five plus in the United States. Washington, DC: US Department of Commerce, Bureau of the Census; 1996.
5. National Research Council. The aging population in the twenty-first century: statistics for health policy. Washington, DC: National Academies Press; 1988.
6. West LA, Cole S, Goodkind D, et al. 65+ in the United States: 2010. Washington, DC: US Census Bureau; 2014.
7. He W, Sengupta M, Velkoff VA, et al. 65+ in the United States: 2005. Princeton (NJ): Citeseer; 2005.
8. US Department of Health and Human Services. Multiple chronic conditions—a strategic framework: optimum health and quality of life for individuals with multiple chronic conditions, 2. Washington, DC: US Department of Health and Human Services; 2010.
9. Ward BW, Schiller JS, Goodman RA. Multiple chronic conditions among US adults: a 2012 update. Prev Chronic Dis 2014;11:130389.
10. Centers for Disease Control and Prevention (CDC). Chronic disease prevention and health promotion. 2016. Available at: http://www.cdc.gov/chronicdisease/index.htm. Accessed March 15, 2018.
11. Gerteis J, Izrael D, Deitz D, et al. Multiple chronic conditions chartbook. Rockville (MD): Agency for Healthcare Research and Quality; 2014.
12. Lochner KA, Goodman RA, Posner S, et al. Multiple chronic conditions among Medicare beneficiaries: state-level variations in prevalence, utilization, and cost, 2011. Medicare Medicaid Res Rev 2013;3(3) [pii:mmrr.003.03.b02].
13. Levit K, Wier L, Stranges E, et al. HCUP facts and figures: statistics on hospital-based care in the United States, 2007. Rockville (MD): Agency for Healthcare Research and Quality; 2009.
14. Hartman M, Martin AB, Espinosa N, et al. National health care spending in 2016: spending and enrollment growth slow after initial coverage expansions. Health Affairs 2017;37(1):150–60.
15. Nardi M, French E, Jones JB, et al. Medical spending of the US elderly. Fiscal Studies 2016;37(3–4):717–47.
16. Centers for Disease Control and Prevention. Web-based injury statistics query and reporting system (WISQARS) [online]. National Center for Injury Prevention and Control, CDC (producer); 2016a. Available at: http://www.cdc.gov/injury/wisqars/index.html. Accessed March 21, 2018.
17. Hodgson TA, Cohen AJ. Medical expenditures for major diseases, 1995. Health Care Financ Rev 1999;21(2):119.
18. Burns ER, Stevens JA, Lee R. The direct costs of fatal and non-fatal falls among older adults—United States. J Safety Res 2016;58:99–103.

19. Stevens JA, Corso PS, Finkelstein EA, et al. The costs of fatal and non-fatal falls among older adults. Inj Prev 2006;12(5):290–5.
20. Rhee P, Joseph B, Pandit V, et al. Increasing trauma deaths in the United States. Ann Surg 2014;260(1):13–21.
21. Hamilton BE, Hoyert DL, Martin JA, et al. Annual summary of vital statistics: 2010–2011. Pediatrics 2013;131(3):548–58.
22. Faul M, Xu L, Wald M, et al. Centers for Disease Control and Prevention. Atlanta (GA): National Center for Injury Prevention and Control; 2010. p. 2–70.
23. Centers for Disease Control and Prevention (CDC), National Center for Injury Prevention and Control. Web-based Injury Statistics Query and Reporting (WISQARS); 2010. Available at: http://www.cdc.gov/injury/wisqars/index.html. Accessed March 20, 2018.
24. Rubenstein LZ. Falls in older people: epidemiology, risk factors and strategies for prevention. Age Ageing 2006;35(suppl_2):ii37–41.
25. Centers for Disease Control and Prevention (CDC). CDC fact sheet–older adult drivers: get the facts. Atlanta (GA): Centers for Disease Control and Prevention; 2013.
26. Massie DL. Analysis of accident rates by age, gender, and time of day based on the 1990 Nationwide personal transportation survey. Final report. Ann Arbor (MI): The University of Michigan Transportation Research Institute; 1993.
27. Federal Highway Administration. Highway statistics 2015. 2015. Available at: https://www.fhwa.dot.gov/policyinformation/statistics/2015/dl20.cfm. Accessed March 20, 2018.
28. Sooryanarayana R, Choo W-Y, Hairi NN. A review on the prevalence and measurement of elder abuse in the community. Trauma Violence Abuse 2013;14(4): 316–25.
29. Anthony EK, Lehning AJ, Austin MJ, et al. Assessing elder mistreatment: instrument development and implications for adult protective services. J Gerontol Soc Work 2009;52(8):815–36.
30. National Center on Elder Abuse. The 2004 survey of state adult protective services: Abuse of adults 60 years of age and older; 2006. Available at: https://ncea.acl.gov/resources/docs/archive/APS-Adults-60plus-FactSheet-2006.pdf. Accessed March 23, 2018.
31. Jackson SL, Hafemeister TL. Enhancing the safety of elderly victims after the close of an APS investigation. J Interpers Violence 2013;28(6):1223–39.
32. Johannesen M, LoGiudice D. Elder abuse: a systematic review of risk factors in community-dwelling elders. Age Ageing 2013;42(3):292–8.
33. Morris JA, Mackenzie EJ, Damiano AM, et al. Mortality in trauma patients. J Trauma 1990;30:1476–82.
34. Lustenberger T, Inaba K, Schnüriger B, et al. Gunshot injuries in the elderly: patterns and outcomes. A national trauma databank analysis. World J Surg 2011; 35(3):528–34.
35. Centers for Disease Control and Prevention (CDC). National center for injury prevention and control. Suicide. Facts at a glance. Atlanta (GA): Centers for Disease Control and Prevention; 2008.
36. Etzioni DA, Liu JH, Maggard MA, et al. The aging population and its impact on the surgery workforce. Ann Surg 2003;238(2):170.
37. Reiss R, Deutsch AA. Emergency abdominal procedures in patients above 70. J Gerontol 1985;40(2):154–8.
38. Horattas MC, Guyton DP, Wu D. A reappraisal of appendicitis in the elderly. Am J Surg 1990;160(3):291–3.

39. Buckius MT, McGrath B, Monk J, et al. Changing epidemiology of acute appendicitis in the United States: study period 1993–2008. J Surg Res 2012;175(2): 185–90.
40. Bingener J, Richards ML, Schwesinger WH, et al. Laparoscopic cholecystectomy for elderly patients: gold standard for golden years? Arch Surg 2003;138(5): 531–6.
41. Borzellino G, De Manzoni G, Ricci F, et al. Emergency cholecystostomy and subsequent cholecystectomy for acute gallstone cholecystitis in the elderly. Br J Surg 1999;86(12):1521–5.
42. Flegal KM, Kit BK, Orpana H, et al. Association of all-cause mortality with overweight and obesity using standard body mass index categories: a systematic review and meta-analysis. JAMA 2013;309(1):71–82.
43. Colquitt JL, Pickett K, Loveman E, et al. Surgery for weight loss in adults. Cochrane Database Syst Rev 2014;(8):CD003641.
44. Kizy S, Jahansouz C, Downey MC, et al. National trends in bariatric surgery 2012–2015: demographics, procedure selection, readmissions, and cost. Obes Surg 2017;27(11):2933–9.
45. Mokdad AH, Serdula MK, Dietz WH, et al. The spread of the obesity epidemic in the United States, 1991-1998. JAMA 1999;282(16):1519–22.
46. Mokdad AH, Bowman BA, Ford ES, et al. The continuing epidemics of obesity and diabetes in the United States. JAMA 2001;286(10):1195–200.
47. Wallace JI, Schwartz RS. Involuntary weight loss in elderly outpatients: recognition, etiologies, and treatment. Clin Geriatr Med 1997;13(4):717–35.
48. Habermann EB, Durham SB, Dorman R, et al. Trends in bariatric surgery in Medicare beneficiaries. Data Points # 17 (prepared by the University of Minnesota DEcIDE Center, under Contract No. HHSA290201000013I). Rockville (MD): Agency for Healthcare Research and Quality; 2012.
49. Etzioni DA, Starnes VA. The epidemiology and economics of cardiothoracic surgery in the elderly. Cardiothoracic surgery in the elderly. New York: Springer; 2011. p. 5–24.
50. Cram P, Lu X, Kates SL, et al. Total knee arthroplasty volume, utilization, and outcomes among Medicare beneficiaries, 1991-2010. JAMA 2012;308(12):1227–36.
51. Yoshihara H, Yoneoka D. Trends in the incidence and in-hospital outcomes of elective major orthopaedic surgery in patients eighty years of age and older in the United States from 2000 to 2009. J Bone Joint Surg Am 2014;96(14):1185–91.
52. Antoniadis A, Ulrich NH, Schmid S, et al. Decompression surgery for lumbar spinal canal stenosis in octogenarians; a single center experience of 121 consecutive patients. Br J Neurosurg 2017;31(1):67–71.
53. Schwab F, Dubey A, Gamez L, et al. Adult scoliosis: prevalence, SF-36, and nutritional parameters in an elderly volunteer population. Spine 2005;30(9):1082–5.
54. Ciol MA, Deyo RA, Howell E, et al. An assessment of surgery for spinal stenosis: time trends, geographic variations, complications, and reoperations. J Am Geriatr Soc 1996;44(3):285–90.
55. Deyo RA, Gray DT, Kreuter W, et al. United States trends in lumbar fusion surgery for degenerative conditions. Spine 2005;30(12):1441–5.
56. Deyo RA, Mirza SK, Martin BI, et al. Trends, major medical complications, and charges associated with surgery for lumbar spinal stenosis in older adults. JAMA 2010;303(13):1259–65.
57. Frontera JA, De Los Reyes K, Gordon E, et al. Trend in outcome and financial impact of subdural hemorrhage. Neurocrit Care 2011;14(2):260–6.

58. Miranda LB, Braxton E, Hobbs J, et al. Chronic subdural hematoma in the elderly: not a benign disease. J Neurosurg 2011;114(1):72–6.
59. Balser D, Farooq S, Mehmood T, et al. Actual and projected incidence rates for chronic subdural hematomas in United States Veterans Administration and civilian populations. J Neurosurg 2015;123(5):1209–15.

Frailty and Prognostication in Geriatric Surgery and Trauma

Cathy A. Maxwell, PhD, RN[a],*, Mayur B. Patel, MD, MPH[b],
Luis C. Suarez-Rodriguez, MD[b], Richard S. Miller, MD[b]

KEYWORDS

- Frailty • Physical frailty • Cognitive frailty • Intrinsic capacity • Geriatric trauma
- Geriatric surgery • Prognostication • Frailty screening

KEY POINTS

- Frailty is a state of vulnerability to stressors (ie, injury) that increases the risk of adverse events, disability, and decline.
- Theoretic constructs for frailty include a phenotype, cumulative deficit model, and a new term, intrinsic capacity.
- Frailty screening is imperative for geriatric trauma and surgical patients.
- The development of prognostic instruments specific to trauma and surgery is an emerging and nascent science.

Frailty is a state of vulnerability to internal and external stressors that increases the risk of adverse events, disability, and decline.[1-3] The past decade has seen an exponential increase in frailty research that integrates frailty measures into clinical practice models. Progress in understanding frailty as a biological process at the cellular and molecular levels has led to a realization of the importance of including frailty measures and/or variables for risk assessment and shared decision making. A growing body of literature within the field of geriatric trauma and surgery has focused on the influence of frailty on patient outcomes. Among geriatric trauma patients, frailty is a predominant predictor of poor outcomes, including discharge to skilled nursing facilities, functional decline, and mortality up to 1-year postinjury.[4,5]

Theoretic constructs for frailty include a phenotype,[6] comprised of physical components, and a cumulative deficit burden model that includes physical, social, functional,

Disclosure: The authors have nothing to disclose.
[a] Vanderbilt University School of Nursing, 461 21st Avenue South, GH 420, Nashville, TN 37240, USA; [b] Division of Trauma and Surgical Critical Care, Vanderbilt University Medical Center, 1211 21st Avenue South, Nashville, TN 37212-1750, USA
* Corresponding author.
E-mail address: Cathy.maxwell@vanderbilt.edu

Clin Geriatr Med 35 (2019) 13–26
https://doi.org/10.1016/j.cger.2018.08.002
0749-0690/19/© 2018 Elsevier Inc. All rights reserved.

geriatric.theclinics.com

and cognitive factors.[7] More recently, frailty is conceptualized within a broader domain of a new term, *intrinsic capacity*, defined as the composite of all the physical and mental capacities of an individual.[8]

This article reviews the concept of frailty and the role of frailty for prognostication among geriatric trauma and surgery patients. First, we discuss models of frailty defined in the scientific literature, emphasizing that frailty is a process of biologic aging. We discuss the importance of screening, assessment, and the inclusion of frailty indices for prognostication. Finally, we discuss best practices for the delivery of prognostic information in acute care settings.

FRAILTY PHENOTYPE

The Fried phenotype model of frailty, derived from the Cardiovascular Health Study (CHS), identifies 5 characteristics that define frailty, including weight loss, self-reported exhaustion, low physical activity, slowness (gait speed), and weakness (grip strength).[6] Within the CHS, baseline evaluations of more than 5000 older participants included self-assessed health, physical function tests, diagnostic procedures, and laboratory tests. Participants were followed for 7 years, leading to the development and operationalization of a frailty phenotype. Frailty was defined as a clinical syndrome in which 3 or more of the 5 characteristics were present. **Table 1** presents each characteristic and the measurement criteria for each. Fried and colleagues[6] demonstrated the predictive value of the phenotype with adverse outcomes of disability, hospitalizations, falls and mortality. Frailty was also strongly associated with cardiovascular disease, pulmonary disease, and diabetes, suggesting common underlying biologic pathways.[9] The Fried study offered the first standardized screening method for risk identification among older adults.[6]

CUMULATIVE DEFICIT FRAILTY INDEX

Derived from the Canadian Study on Health and Aging (CSHA), Rockwood and Mitnitski[7] developed the cumulative deficit model of frailty, or frailty index. Within the CSHA, more than 10,000 older adult participants were followed for 5 years with the aim of describing the epidemiology of cognitive impairment and other health issues associated with aging. The model identified 70 deficits, including signs and symptoms, laboratory values, and disabilities that accumulate in older adults. A frailty index was calculated by dividing the total number of deficits present by the number of variables

| Table 1 | |
| Fried phenotype criteria and measurement indices | |
FP Criteria	Measurement
Weight loss	>10% of unintentional weight loss during the prior year
Weakness	Grip strength <20th percentile
Slowness	Walking time (15 feet): slowest 20% by sex and height
Low level of physical activity	Bottom 20th percentile of calculated kilocalories as measured by the Minnesota Leisure Time Activity Questionnaire
Exhaustion	Self-reported, based on items in the Center for Epidemiologic Studies Depression Scale

Scoring rubric for criteria met: 0, nonfrail; 1–2, prefrail; ≥3, frail.
Data from Fried LP, Tangen CM, Walston J, et al. Frailty in older adults: evidence for a phenotype. J Gerontol A Biol Sci Med Sci 2001;56(3):M146–56.

examined. Modified versions of the frailty index are based on smaller numbers of deficits ranging from 12 to 40 of the original 70.[10–14] **Box 1** lists the original 70 variables included in the model. Rooted within the model was the importance of function and frailty, which led to the development of the Clinical Frailty Scale, a measure of frailty that ranks patients on a 7-point scale from very fit to severely frailty.[15]

SUBCATEGORIES OF FRAILTY

A 2013 consensus conference on frailty identified a subcategory of physical frailty as a distinct entity.[3] Based on the Fried phenotype model, physical frailty was defined as "a medical syndrome with multiple causes and contributors that is, characterized by diminished strength, endurance and reduced physiologic function that increases an individual's vulnerability for developing increased dependency and/or death."[3] Caveats include that (1) not all disabled persons are frail, but frailty can lead to disability, (2) frailty differs from sarcopenia (loss of muscle tissue associated with aging) and is more multifaceted, (3) a diagnosis of frailty should be determined using criteria of well-defined models, and (4) physical frailty differs from multimorbidity.[3]

Cognitive frailty is a subcategory defined as the presence of both physical frailty and cognitive impairment, excluding concurrent Alzheimer dementia or other dementias.[16] Cognitive frailty demonstrates the link between physical function and cognitive functional decline and explains that it may be a precursor of neurodegenerative processes, with the potential for reversibility.[16] Cognitive impairment improves the predictive validity of the frailty phenotype,[17] raising the importance of including cognitive measures in risk assessment.

INTRINSIC CAPACITY

In 2015, the World Health Organization published the World Report on Aging and Health,[18] recommending major shifts in how health policies are formulated and services provided. Emphasizing the evidence that the loss of ability with aging is only loosely associated with chronologic age, functional and cognitive capacity is rooted in events throughout the life course that can be modified to improve health and mitigate decline. Within the World Health Organization report and based on large-scale epidemiologic data, trajectories of physical capacity across the life course were mapped, noting that the range of potential physical functioning is far greater in older age than in younger ages. For example, a 70 year old could have the same physical capacity of a 20 year old, yet another 70 year old may experience significant functional decline. This diversity is not random and reflects a compilation of predictive factors. Healthy aging is defined as "the process of developing and maintaining the functional ability that enables well-being in older age."[18(p28)] Within this framework, the concept of intrinsic capacity emerged, representing the composite of all the physical and mental capacities of an individual.[18]

Within the World Health Organization model, healthy aging is predicated on a longitudinal observation of individuals' trajectories to support preemptive and personalized interventions that enhance capacities and abilities. This approach encourages a transition from reactive medicine toward a more preventive model. An intrinsic capacity framework identifies 5 domains: (1) cognition, (2) psychological (ie, mood and sociality), (3) sensory function (ie, vision, hearing), (4) vitality (bioenergetics, balance between energy intake and energy use), and (5) locomotion (ie, muscular function).[8] **Table 2** presents the 5 domains of intrinsic capacity, along with subdomains of each. The framework provides a model to guide education, research, and practice.

Box 1
Cumulative deficits for frailty index (70 variables from the Canadian Study of health and aging)

- Changes in everyday activities
- Head and neck problems
- Poor muscle tone in neck
- Bradykinesia, facial
- Problems getting dressed
- Problems with bathing
- Problems carrying out personal grooming
- Impaired mobility
- Musculoskeletal problems
- Bradykinesia of the limbs
- Poor muscle tone in limbs
- Poor limb coordination
- Depression (clinical impression)
- Sleep changes
- Restlessness
- Memory changes
- Short-term memory impairment
- Long-term memory impairment
- Changes in general mental functioning
- Onset of cognitive symptoms
- Clouding or delirium
- Paranoid features
- History relevant to cognitive impairment or loss
- Family history relevant to cognitive impairment or loss
- Impaired vibration
- Tremor at rest
- Postural tremor
- Intention tremor
- History of Parkinson's disease
- Family history of degenerative disease
- Seizures, partial complex
- Seizure, generalized
- Syncope or blackouts
- Headache
- Cerebrovascular problems
- History of stroke
- History of diabetes mellitus

- Malignant disease
- Breast problems
- Abdominal problems
- Presence of snout reflex
- Presence of palmomental reflex
- Other medical history
- Poor coordination, trunk
- Poor standing posture
- Irregular gait pattern
- Falls
- Mood problems
- Feeling sad, blue, depressed
- History of depressed mood
- Tiredness all the time
- Arterial hypertension
- Peripheral pulses
- Cardiac problems
- Myocardial infarction
- Arrhythmia
- Congestive heart failure
- Lung problems
- Respiratory problems
- History of thyroid disease
- Thyroid problems
- Skin problems
- Toileting problems
- Bulk difficulties
- Rectal problems
- Urinary incontinence
- Gastrointestinal problems
- Problems cooking
- Sucking problems
- Problems going out alone

Scoring rubric: Number of deficits identified divided by total number of deficits assessed (range, 0–1).
Data from Mitnitski AB, Mogilner AJ, Rockwood K. Accumulation of deficits as a proxy measure of aging. ScientificWorldJournal 2001;1:323–36.

The concept of intrinsic capacity focuses on residual biological reserves that explain the development of frailty. Dysfunction in multiple physiologic systems contributes to the development of frailty and multiple chronic disease states, including vascular disease, diabetes, pulmonary disease, depression, and congestive heart failure.

Table 2
Domains comprising intrinsic capacity with examples of measurement indices

Cognition	Locomotion	Psychological	Vitality	Sensory
• Memory	• Balance	• Mood	• Bioenergetics	• Vision
• Executive function	• Strength	• Emotional	• Hormonal function	• Hearing
• Visuospatial	• Endurance	vitality	• Cardiopulmonary	
perception	• Gait		function	

Data from World Health Organization. World report on ageing and health. Available at: http://www.who.int/ageing/publications/world-report-2015/en/. Accessed February 18, 2017.

Physiologic systems thought to drive late life vulnerability and frailty include a dysregulated sympathetic nervous system, the innate immune system, and the hypothalamic–pituitary–adrenal axis.[19] Additionally, age-related changes in mitochondrial function are thought to contribute to chronic inflammatory pathways,[20] neurodegenerative disorders,[21] and pulmonary and cardiac fibrosis,[22] as well as sarcopenia.[23,24] These biological foundations highlight the importance of including frailty measures for risk adjustment in studies, as well as prognostication models with older adults, because their omission could lead to inaccurate and erroneous findings.[25,26]

FRAILTY SCREENING AND PROGNOSTICATION

The theoretic underpinnings of frailty emphasize the importance of screening older adults to determine baseline physical and mental capacities for the purpose of risk assessment, preventive intervention, and anticipatory care related to the eventual end of life. Among geriatric trauma and surgery patients, obtaining baseline frailty and cognitive measures is essential for accurate prognostication. **Table 3** provides a list of useful screening instruments (with descriptions) for acute care settings. Instrument choice should be guided by (1) predictive ability of the outcome of interest (eg, mortality, adverse events), (2) predictive response to interventions (eg, ABCDEF bundle, mobilization protocols), (3) support of biological causative theory, and (4) simplicity of use.[27]

Among geriatric trauma and surgical populations, prognostication is influenced by not only the underlying biological basis of frailty, but also by the severity of injury, as well as the interventions delivered during the acute care phase. The development of prognostic instruments specific to trauma and surgery is an emerging and nascent science. To date, 5 prediction/prognostic models exist, and 3 have been used in studies other than the derivation study. The following section describes the development of each model and other studies that have used the instrument.

TRAUMA-SPECIFIC FRAILTY INDEX

The Trauma-Specific Frailty Index (TSFI) is a 15-variable scale assessing comorbidities and prehospital factors that predicts discharge disposition to either home/rehabilitation or to unfavorable dispositions (skilled nursing facilities, death).[10] Fifteen variables among 50 original frailty index deficits were selected based on univariate associations with discharge dispositions among 100 geriatric trauma patients. Selected variables were subsequently tested in a representative sample of 200 patients admitted to a level I trauma center over a 2-year period.[10] Variable categories that comprise the TSFI include comorbid conditions, daily activities, health attitudes, function, and nutrition. Fifteen items are scored and totaled. The score is then divided by

Table 3
Frailty screening instruments

Instrument	Number of Items	Description of Content
Edmonton Frailty Scale[52]	11	Nine domains (cognition, general health, functional independence, social support, medication use, nutrition, mood, continence, functional performance) scored from 0 to 2
Tilburg Frailty Indicator[53]	25	Demographic data; domains: physical, psychological and social components of frailty
PRISMA-7[54]	7	Yes/no format; domains: age, sex, health limitations (n = 2), need for assistance (n = 2), use of assistive devices
Groningen Frailty Indicator[55]	15	Yes/no format; domains: mobility, vision, hearing, nutrition, comorbidity, cognition, psychosocial, physical fitness
Vulnerable Elders Survey[56]	13	Domains: age, self-rated health, common physical activities, activities of daily living
Identification of Seniors at Risk[57]	6	Yes/no format; domains: need for assistance, past hospitalizations, vision, memory, number of medications
Short Physical Performance Battery[58]	3	Domains: balance, gait speed, chair stand
Rapid Screening Tools		
FRAIL Questionnaire[59]	5	Yes/no format; fatigue, resistance, ambulation, illnesses, loss of weight
Clinical Frailty Scale[15]	NA	9 point scale from very fit (n = 1) to terminally ill (n = 9); silhouettes and descriptions
Gerontopole Frailty Screening Tool[60]	6	Yes/no format; living arrangements, weight loss, fatigue, mobility, memory loss, gait speed

the number of items, resulting in a TSFI score (range, 0–1). The study determined that frail patients with a TSFI of greater than 0.27 were more likely to have an unfavorable discharge disposition.[10] The study did not examine postdischarge outcomes, including functional decline, readmissions to acute care, quality of life, or delayed mortality. Since the development of the TSFI, subsequent studies have reported associations between the TSFI and failure to rescue,[28] trauma-related readmissions,[29] and repeat falls.[29]

GERIATRIC TRAUMA OUTCOME SCORE

The Geriatric Trauma Outcome Score (GTOS) was developed as a prognostic tool for mortality during the index hospitalization. Developed retrospectively from trauma registry data on 3841 geriatric trauma patients over 13 years, the GTOS is composed of 3 variables: (1) age, (2) Injury Severity Score × 2.5, and (3) blood transfusion during the first 24 hours of hospitalization (22 points).[30] Based on logistic regression models, the predicted probability of death during hospitalization ranges from 1% (GTOS of 60) to 99% (GTOS of >290). A nomogram is available for comparison of the GTOS score to the percent probability of mortality. For example, an 82-year-old patients (82 points) with and Injury Severity Score of 12 (36 points) who received packed cells within 24 hours of admission (22 points) would have a GTOS of 140 or a predicted probability of in-hospital mortality of approximately 20%. The derivation study was later validated in a sample of geriatric trauma patients from 4 level I trauma centers (N = 18,282) that reported similar findings.[31] Subsequent studies examined the predictive capacity of GTOS for other outcomes. Cook and colleagues[32] reported moderate predictive accuracy for unfavorable discharge (skilled nursing facility, long-term acute care, hospice). Ahl and colleagues[33] reported that although the GTOS was accurate in predicting in-patient mortality, the model was not able to predict 1-year mortality.

PALLIATIVE PERFORMANCE SCALE

The Palliative Performance Scale (PPS) is a modification of the Karnofsky Performance Scale,[34] which was developed for predicting patients' ability to survive chemotherapy. The PPS is a reliable and validated tool[35] that can be used in any clinical setting for describing a person's current functional level. Ten levels of function are described across 5 domains: (1) ambulation ability (full, reduced, mainly sit or lie, bed bound, death), (2) activity level (normal activity and work, normal activity with effort, unable normal, unable hobby or housework, unable to do most or any activity), (3) self-care ability (full, occasional assistance, considerable assistance, mainly assistance, total care), (4) oral intake (normal, reduced, minimal to sips, mouth care only), and (5) level of consciousness (full, confusion, drowsy, coma). Each level is associated with a predicted probability (%) of survival. Among the geriatric trauma population, McGreevy and colleagues[36] reported that the PPS identified unmet palliative care needs and was an independent predictor of in-patient mortality, poor functional outcomes, and discharge to dependent care. Subsequent studies in other older populations also predicted functional decline[37] and 6-month survival.[38]

OTHER INSTRUMENTS

Two additional prognostic models have been developed for the populations of interest, including a tool to predict postoperative complications among emergency general surgery patients[39] and a tool that predicts functional decline/mortality among geriatric trauma patients.[40] To our knowledge, follow-up validation studies have not been conducted for either instrument. Jokar and colleagues[39] developed an Emergency General Surgery Frailty Index using the same methodology used for the development of the TSFI. The Emergency General Surgery Frailty Index is composed of 15 variables that assess the frailty status of patients undergoing emergency surgery. The Emergency General Surgery Frailty Index was found to be an independent predictor of postoperative complications, including pneumonia, sepsis, urinary tract infection, and other complications. In a later study, Jeffery and colleagues[40] developed a prediction model from a prior study of 188 geriatric trauma patients evaluating outcomes at 4 time points after injury (1 month, 3 months, 6 months, 1 year). Using variables from the original prospective study, the investigators identified 6 variables most predictive of functional decline and mortality. A nomogram of the predictors was developed and found to be highly accurate ($R^2 = 0.96$) for clinical prediction of 1-year mortality. The relative importance of predictors from largest to smallest were Life Space Assessment score, Vulnerable Elder Survey score, Injury Severity Score, Barthel Index (disability) score, comorbidity index, first principal component (statistical procedure), and the AD8 Dementia Screen score.[40]

In summary, relatively few studies exist to guide clinicians in the prognostication of geriatric trauma or surgery patients. Fundamentally, studies should seek to explain the relative importance of both injury-specific and aging-specific interventions in the face of varying injury severity and preadmission factors such as cognitive and functional status. **Table 4** compares the current validated models (TSFI, GTOS, PPS) according to descriptions, variables, and predicted outcomes. Of note, online prognostication tools, developed from secondary analyses of large data of older adults, are also available to facilitate care. These include ePrognosis[41] and the American College of Surgeons National Surgery Quality Improvement Program Surgical Risk Calculator.[42] Future research is needed for the validation of existing models and the development of new models, as well as to determine optimal use of these models in clinical practice.

Table 4
Prognostication tools for geriatric trauma and surgery: Predictive variables and outcomes

Trauma-Specific Frailty Index	Geriatric Trauma Outcome Score	Palliative Performance Scale
Cancer history:	Age	Ambulation
• Yes/no	Injury severity	• Full
Coronary heart disease	• ISS × 2.5	• Reduced
• MI (1); CABG (0.75); PCI (0.50);	Packed red blood cells	• Mainly sit/lie
Meds (0.25); No meds (0)	• Transfused ≤24 h of	• Totally bed bound
Dementia	admission (22 points)	Activity and evidence of disease
• Severe (1); moderate (0.50);	Total score (range,	• Normal activity to inability to
mild (0.25); none (0)	60–295)	do any activity
Help with grooming (Y/N)		• No evidence of disease to
Help managing money (Y/N)		Extensive disease
Help household work (Y/N)		Self-care
Help toileting (Y/N)		• Full
Help walking		• Occasional assistance
• Wheelchair (1); walker (0.75);		• Considerable assistance
cane (0.25); none (0)		• Mainly assistance
Feel less useful		• Total care
• Most of the time (1);		Intake
sometimes (0.50); never (0)		• Normal
Feel sad		• Reduced
• Most of the time (1);		• Minimal to sips
sometimes (0.50); never (0)		• Mouth care only
Feel effort to do everything		Consciousness level
• Most of the time (1);		• Full
sometimes (0.50); never (0)		• Confusion
Falls		• Drowsy with or without
• Most of the time (1);		confusion
sometimes (.50); never (0)		
Feel lonely		
• Most of the time (1);		
sometimes (0.50); never (0)		
Sexually active (Y/N)		
Nutrition, albumin		
• <3 (1); >3 (0)		
Outcomes:	Outcomes:	Outcomes:
Discharge disposition (cutoff: 0.27, favorable [home, rehabilitation] vs unfavorable [death, long-term care facility])	Percent probability of in-patient mortality (range, 1% [score of 60] to 99% [score of >290])	Mortality/survival, poor functional outcomes, discharge to dependent care (range, 100% [no limitations to 0% [death]).

Abbreviations: CABG, coronary artery bypass graft; ISS, Injury Severity Score; MI, myocardial infarction; PCI, percutaneous coronary intervention; Y/N, yes/no.

COMMUNICATION OF PROGNOSTIC INFORMATION IN ACUTE CARE SETTINGS

Studies show that intervening events (falls, injury, hospitalizations) highly influence the disabling process in frail older adults by accelerating functional decline.[43,44] Relatedly, exposure to personal critical illness provides a window of opportunity for prognostic discussions and shared decision making that may lead to behavior change, enhanced quality of life, or acceptance of the approaching end of life.[45] When patients and families have a poor understanding of prognosis, decision making and elicitation of preferences and values is hindered.[46] In older adults, this facto is particularly important because discussions can occur at multiple stages in the frailty trajectory to encourage decision making aimed at 3 points: primary prevention, delay of frailty progression, and facilitation of advance care planning and palliative care. The inclusion of prognostic information is a best practice in establishing goals of care and early (vs late) discussions are recommended to achieve the full impact of care processes.[47] Studies show that older patients want to be fully informed about their prognosis,[47,48] although physicians are often reluctant to engage in discussions until death is imminent.[49]

Key stakeholders and experts in prognostic communication offer recommendations to facilitate the delivery of prognostic information to older adults and family caregivers. Cooper and colleagues[50] convened an interdisciplinary advisory panel of national leaders and proposed a communication framework to facilitate goal-concordant care for seriously ill older adults with surgical emergencies. Core communication components included the conveyance of prognostic information that included assessment of baseline functional performance (ie, frailty status) and advanced chronic conditions. The panel urged recognition that communication is a requisite clinical skill for delivering high-quality surgical care and that conversations should occur within the context of the patient's total care versus surgical goal.

Anderson and colleagues[51] interviewed 118 key stakeholders from multiple disciplines to determine perspectives on how prognostic information should be conveyed in critical illness. Recommendations included honest disclosure of prognostic information, emotional support, tailoring suggestions to the individual patient and family, and verifying that the patient and family understand the material presented to them. Of particular importance is the recognition that prognostic communication should occur as an iterative process. Difficult discussions about aging, frailty, and the approaching end of life require time to reflect and adapt, while balancing expectations with realistic forms of hope.[48] Staged discussions provide the opportunity for patients and caregivers to ponder information, adapt, and formulate priorities that are most meaningful to them. Within the field of geriatric trauma and surgery, the delivery of prognostic information should be a prime area of focus for education, research, and clinical care to improve patient outcomes, including health care use, cost of care, and behavior change (eg, lifestyle, fall prevention).

SUMMARY

Frailty poses a public health crisis for an aging society and is particularly relevant to the geriatric trauma and surgery populations. It is imperative that trauma centers throughout the United States integrate frailty screening procedures into daily clinical workflow to enhance quality of care. Recommendations include the (1) development of hospital-specific practice management guidelines for frailty screening and initiation of geriatric palliative care, (2) use of frailty screening measures for risk assessment/adjustment in quality improvement efforts, and (3) incorporation of frailty measures into trauma registry data for research and national reporting (ie, National Trauma Data Bank). Although daunting, these tasks are achievable through a multidisciplinary approach aimed at education and implementation of procedures integrated into established workflows. The use of validated screening instruments with low response burden for both patients and providers (eg, FRAIL questionnaire, Clinical Frailty Scale) will help to ensure success, along with identification of clinical leaders to champion rollouts and ongoing efforts.

This article provides an overview of the concept of frailty, highlighting a pressing need for providers to not only understand the concept, but also incorporate best practices for frailty assessment and optimal communication of prognostic information to patients and families. The time is now for transition from theory to practice to improve outcomes and advance policies that facilitate optimal care of the geriatric patient.

REFERENCES

1. Clegg A, Young J. The frailty syndrome. Clin Med (Lond) 2011;11(1):72–5.
2. Lang PO, Michel JP, Zekry D. Frailty syndrome: a transitional state in a dynamic process. Gerontology 2009;55(5):539–49.
3. Morley JE, Vellas B, van Kan GA, et al. Frailty consensus: a call to action. J Am Med Dir Assoc 2013;14(6):392–7.
4. Joseph B, Pandit V, Zangbar B, et al. Superiority of frailty over age in predicting outcomes among geriatric trauma patients: a prospective analysis. JAMA Surg 2014;149(8):766–72.
5. Maxwell CA, Mion LC, Mukherjee K, et al. Preinjury physical frailty and cognitive impairment among geriatric trauma patients determine postinjury functional recovery and survival. J Trauma Acute Care Surg 2016;80(2):195–203.
6. Fried LP, Tangen CM, Walston J, et al. Frailty in older adults: evidence for a phenotype. J Gerontol A Biol Sci Med Sci 2001;56(3):M146–56.
7. Mitnitski AB, Mogilner AJ, Rockwood K. Accumulation of deficits as a proxy measure of aging. ScientificWorldJournal 2001;1:323–36.
8. Cesari M, Araujo de Carvalho I, Amuthavalli Thiyagarajan J, et al. Evidence for the domains supporting the construct of intrinsic capacity. J Gerontol A Biol Sci Med Sci 2018. [Epub ahead of print].
9. Auyeung TW, Lee JS, Leung J, et al. The selection of a screening test for frailty identification in community-dwelling older adults. J Nutr Health Aging 2014; 18(2):199–203.
10. Joseph B, Pandit V, Zangbar B, et al. Validating trauma-specific frailty index for geriatric trauma patients: a prospective analysis. J Am Coll Surg 2014;219(1): 10–7.e1.
11. Mitnitski AB, Song X, Rockwood K. The estimation of relative fitness and frailty in community-dwelling older adults using self-report data. J Gerontol A Biol Sci Med Sci 2004;59(6):M627–32.
12. Yu P, Song X, Shi J, et al. Frailty and survival of older Chinese adults in urban and rural areas: results from the Beijing Longitudinal Study of Aging. Arch Gerontol Geriatr 2012;54(1):3–8.
13. Adams P, Ghanem T, Stachler R, et al. Frailty as a predictor of morbidity and mortality in inpatient head and neck surgery. JAMA Otolaryngol Head Neck Surg 2013;139(8):783–9.
14. Hoogendijk EO, Theou O, Rockwood K, et al. Development and validation of a frailty index in the longitudinal aging study Amsterdam. Aging Clin Exp Res 2017;29(5):927–33.
15. Rockwood K, Song X, MacKnight C, et al. A global clinical measure of fitness and frailty in elderly people. CMAJ 2005;173(5):489–95.

16. Kelaiditi E, Cesari M, Canevelli M, et al. Cognitive frailty: rational and definition from an (IANA/IAGG) international consensus group. J Nutr Health Aging 2013; 17(9):726–34.

17. Ávila-Funes JA, Amieva H, Barberger-Gateau P, et al. Cognitive impairment improves the predictive validity of the phenotype of frailty for adverse health outcomes: the three-city study. J Am Geriatr Soc 2009;57(3):453–61.

18. World Health Organization (WHO). World report on ageing and health. Geneva (Switzerland): World Health Organization; 2015. Available at: http://www.who.int/ageing/publications/world-report-2015/en/. Accessed February 18, 2017.

19. Walston JD. Connecting age-related biological decline to frailty and late-life vulnerability. In: Fielding RA, Sieber C, Vellas B, editors. Frailty: pathophysiology, phenotype and patient care, vol. 83. Karger Publishers; 2015. p. 1–10.

20. Kaminskyy VO, Zhivotovsky B. Free radicals in cross talk between autophagy and apoptosis. Antioxid Redox Signal 2014;21(1):86–102.

21. Ghavami S, Shojaei S, Yeganeh B, et al. Autophagy and apoptosis dysfunction in neurodegenerative disorders. Prog Neurobiol 2014;112:24–49.

22. Biernacka A, Frangogiannis NG. Aging and cardiac fibrosis. Aging Dis 2011;2(2): 158.

23. Akki A, Yang H, Gupta A, et al. Skeletal muscle ATP kinetics are impaired in frail mice. Age (Dordr) 2014;36(1):21–30.

24. Distefano G, Standley RA, Zhang X, et al. Physical activity unveils the relationship between mitochondrial energetics, muscle quality, and physical function in older adults. J Cachexia Sarcopenia Muscle 2018;9(2):279–94.

25. Shamliyan T, Talley KM, Ramakrishnan R, et al. Association of frailty with survival: a systematic literature review. Ageing Res Rev 2013;12(2):719–36.

26. Kautter J, Ingber M, Pope GC. Medicare risk adjustment for the frail elderly. Health Care Financ Rev 2008;30(2):83.

27. Clegg A, Young J, Iliffe S, et al. Frailty in elderly people. Lancet 2013;381(9868): 752–62.

28. Joseph B, Phelan H, Hassan A, et al. The impact of frailty on failure-to-rescue in geriatric trauma patients: a prospective study. J Trauma Acute Care Surg 2016; 81(6):1150–5.

29. Joseph B, Jokar TO, Hassan A, et al. Redefining the association between old age and poor outcomes after trauma: the impact of frailty syndrome. J Trauma Acute Care Surg 2017;82(3):575–81.

30. Zhao FZ, Wolf SE, Nakonezny PA, et al. Estimating geriatric mortality after injury using age, injury severity, and performance of a transfusion: the Geriatric Trauma Outcome Score. J Palliat Med 2015;18(8):677–81.

31. Cook AC, Joseph B, Inaba K, et al. Multicenter external validation of the geriatric trauma outcome score: a study by the prognostic assessment of life and limitations after trauma in the elderly (PALLIATE) consortium. J Trauma Acute Care Surg 2016;80(2):204–9.

32. Cook AC, Joseph B, Mohler MJ, et al. Validation of a geriatric trauma prognosis calculator: a PAL Li. ATE consortium study. J Am Geriatr Soc 2017;65(10):2302–7.

33. Ahl R, Phelan HA, Dogan S, et al. Predicting in-hospital and 1-year mortality in geriatric trauma patients using Geriatric Trauma Outcome Score. J Am Coll Surg 2017;224(3):264–9.

34. Karnofsky DA, Abelmann WH, Craver LF, et al. The use of the nitrogen mustards in the palliative treatment of carcinoma. With particular reference to bronchogenic carcinoma. Cancer 1948;1(4):634–56.

35. Ho F, Lau F, Downing MG, et al. A reliability and validity study of the Palliative Performance Scale. BMC Palliat Care 2008;7(1):10.
36. McGreevy C, Bryczkowski S, Pentakota SR, et al. Unmet palliative care needs in elderly trauma patients: can the palliative performance scale help close the gap? Am J Surg 2017;213(4):778–84.
37. de Medeiros RB, Stamm AMNF, Moritz RD, et al. Serial palliative performance scale assessment in a university general hospital: a pilot study. J Palliat Med 2018;21(6):842–5.
38. Seedhom AE, Kamal NN. The palliative performance scale predicts survival among emergency department patients, Minia, Egypt. Indian J Palliat Care 2017;23(4):368.
39. Jokar TO, Ibraheem K, Rhee P, et al. Emergency general surgery specific frailty index: a validation study. J Trauma Acute Care Surg 2016;81(2):254–60.
40. Jeffery AD, Dietrich MS, Maxwell CA. Predicting 1-year disability and mortality of injured older adults. Arch Gerontol Geriatr 2018;75:191–6.
41. University of California at San Francisco. ePrognosis. Available at: https://eprognosis.ucsf.edu/index.php. Accessed February 15, 2018.
42. American College of Surgeons. NSQIP Surgical Risk Calculator. 2018. Available at: https://riskcalculator.facs.org/RiskCalculator/index.jsp. Accessed February 15, 2018.
43. Gill TM, Murphy TE, Gahbauer EA, et al. The course of disability before and after a serious fall injury. JAMA Intern Med 2013;173(19):1780–6.
44. Gill TM, Gahbauer EA, Han L, et al. The role of intervening hospital admissions on trajectories of disability in the last year of life: prospective cohort study of older people. BMJ 2015;350:h2361.
45. Ernecoff NC, Keane CR, Albert SM. Health behavior change in advance care planning: an agent-based model. BMC Public Health 2016;16(1):193.
46. Wagner GJ, Riopelle D, Steckart J, et al. Provider communication and patient understanding of life-limiting illness and their relationship to patient communication of treatment preferences. J Pain Symptom Manage 2010;39(3):527–34.
47. Bernacki RE, Block SD. Communication about serious illness care goals: a review and synthesis of best practices. JAMA Intern Med 2014;174(12):1994–2003.
48. Parker SM, Clayton JM, Hancock K, et al. A systematic review of prognostic/end-of-life communication with adults in the advanced stages of a life-limiting illness: patient/caregiver preferences for the content, style, and timing of information. J Pain Symptom Manage 2007;34(1):81–93.
49. Hoff L, Hermerén G. Identifying challenges to communicating with patients about their imminent death. J Clin Ethics 2014;25(4):296–306.
50. Cooper Z, Koritsanszky LA, Cauley CE, et al. Recommendations for best communication practices to facilitate goal-concordant care for seriously ill older patients with emergency surgical conditions. Ann Surg 2016;263(1):1–6.
51. Anderson WG, Cimino JW, Ernecoff NC, et al. A multicenter study of key stakeholders' perspectives on communicating with surrogates about prognosis in intensive care units. Ann Am Thorac Soc 2015;12(2):142–52.
52. Rolfson DB, Majumdar SR, Tsuyuki RT, et al. Validity and reliability of the Edmonton frail scale. Age Ageing 2006;35(5):526–9.
53. Gobbens RJ, van Assen MA, Luijkx KG, et al. The Tilburg frailty indicator: psychometric properties. J Am Med Dir Assoc 2010;11(5):344–55.
54. Raîche M, Hébert R, Dubois MF. PRISMA-7: a case-finding tool to identify older adults with moderate to severe disabilities. Arch Gerontol Geriatr 2008;47(1):9–18.

55. Steverink N, Slaets J, Schuurmans H, et al. Measuring frailty. Development and testing of the Groningen frailty indicator (GFI). Gerontologist 2001;41(1):236.
56. Saliba D, Elliott M, Rubenstein LZ, et al. The Vulnerable Elders Survey: a tool for identifying vulnerable older people in the community. J Am Geriatr Soc 2001; 49(12):1691–9.
57. Salvi F, Morichi V, Grilli A, et al. Screening for frailty in elderly emergency department patients by using the Identification of Seniors at Risk (ISAR). J Nutr Health Aging 2012;16(4):313–8.
58. Guralnik JM, Simonsick EM, Ferrucci L, et al. A short physical performance battery assessing lower extremity function: association with self-reported disability and prediction of mortality and nursing home admission. J Gerontol 1994; 49(2):M85–94.
59. Morley JE, Malmstrom T, Miller D. A simple frailty questionnaire (FRAIL) predicts outcomes in middle aged African Americans. J Nutr Health Aging 2012;16(7): 601–8.
60. Vellas B, Balardy L, Gillette-Guyonnet S, et al. Looking for frailty in community-dwelling older persons: the Gerontopole Frailty Screening Tool (GFST). J Nutr Health Aging 2013;17(7):629–31.

Utilization of Geriatric Consultation and Team-Based Care

Joseph F. Sucher, MD[a],*, Alicia J. Mangram, MD[b],
James K. Dzandu, PhD[c]

KEYWORDS

- Geriatric consultation services • Geriatric wards • Geriatric multidisciplinary teams
- G60 trauma • Comprehensive geriatric assessment • Acute care for elderly
- Geriatric evaluation and management

KEY POINTS

- People in the United States are living longer and, therefore, are at increased risk for adverse events in the acute care setting compared with their younger counterparts.
- Elderly patients' risk of adverse outcomes can be attenuated by early definitive, aggressive, and effective surgical strategies combined with a multidisciplinary team that is focused on the unique needs of the geriatric patient.
- There are multiple models of assessment and delivery of care for geriatric surgical patients. In this review of the literature, and in the authors' unique experience with geriatric trauma care (G60 trauma), the authors believe that a surgeon leader working with a multidisciplinary team provides optimal care with the greatest efficiency and utilization of resources.

INTRODUCTION

Age is an issue of mind over matter. If you don't mind, it doesn't matter.
—(anonymous government researcher c. 1968)

The segment of the American population 65 years and older is expected to nearly double from 37 million people in 2005 to more than 70 million by 2030.[1] The effect is already seen with the percent of inpatient admissions for those older than 65 in the United States having increased "from 43% (2000) to 50% (2013) among all acute

Disclosure: The authors have nothing to disclose.
[a] Valley Surgical Clinics and Acute Care Surgical Specialists, HonorHealth Deer Valley Hospital, 19841 N 27th Avenue, MOB Suite 200, Phoenix, AZ 85027, USA; [b] Valley Surgical Clinics and Acute Care Surgical Specialists, HonorHealth John C Lincoln Hospital, 250 E. Dunlap, Phoenix, AZ 85250, USA; [c] HonorHealth John C Lincoln Hospital, 250 E. Dunlap, Phoenix, AZ 85250, USA
* Corresponding author.
E-mail address: Joseph.Suchermd@honorhealth.com

Clin Geriatr Med 35 (2019) 27–33
https://doi.org/10.1016/j.cger.2018.08.003
0749-0690/19/© 2018 Elsevier Inc. All rights reserved.

care hospitals."[2] Although the family practice and internal medicine disciplines have long cared for the elderly, due in large part to the nature of age-associated increased disease burden, the surgical specialties are now caring for increasing numbers of elderly patients. A significant number of these older patients are cared for by both general surgeons and trauma surgeons. For example, admissions of elderly patients to trauma centers rose from 18% in 2005 to 30% in 2017. Between 2014 and 2017, more than 50% of level 3 trauma center admissions in the authors' trauma system were 60 years old and older. With these statistics in mind, physicians, health care teams, hospitals, health care networks, and payors have been looking for innovative methods to optimize acute and long-term health care delivery for the elderly.

Differences between the elderly and younger adults may seem obvious. For instance, their physiologic reserve and response to injury are different from those in their younger counterparts.[3–10] With age begins an increase in the number of chronic medical conditions. These chronic conditions begin to rise significantly in the fourth decade of life and affect approximately 9 of 10 Americans by the eighth decade.[11] Therefore, it is only reasonable that the initial focus needed to be on identifying those patients at increased risk for complications and/or need for long-term care after discharge. *Frailty* is a term often used to identify patients at increased risk for poor outcome. "Frailty is commonly defined as a state of reduced physiologic capacity and increased susceptibility to disability because of age-related loss of physical, cognitive, social, and physiologic functioning."[12] Multiple studies from the trauma literature have identified frailty as a meaningful way to risk-stratify elderly patients at higher risk for adverse outcomes.[13–18] Other publications from the acute care surgery literature have documented the increased risk of complications, ICU needs, and hospital length of stay in elderly acute care surgery patients.[19–21] These efforts have generally brought about a unique aggressive focus for the care of surgical patients, including "early surgery, immediate mobilization, prevention and management of delirium, pain and malnutrition, as well as an integrated and multidisciplinary approach."[22]

Over the past 3 decades, there has been a tremendous effort in the development, implementation, and evaluation of comprehensive geriatric assessment programs, also known as geriatric evaluation and management (GEM). Comprehensive geriatric asses is often described as a "multidimensional interdisciplinary diagnostic process focused on determining a frail older person's medical, psychological and functional capability in order to develop a coordinated and integrated plan for treatment and long term follow up."[23] As such, a few models have been implemented, including geriatric consultation services, geriatric wards, and geriatric multidisciplinary teams.

GERIATRIC CONSULTATION SERVICES

Wise people understand the need to consult experts. Only fools are confident they know everything.

—Ken Poirot

The geriatrician's expertise lies in a deeper understanding of the aged in regard to age-related changes in physiology, the physical and psychosocial alterations, common impairments in functional status, and the particular challenges of polypharmacy. According to the American Geriatrics Society, the nation requires at least 17,000 geriatricians to meet the needs of the more than 12 million elderly Americans. There are, however, only approximately 7500 certified geriatricians currently in practice. Owing to the small pool of these specialists, it stands to reason that a consultation service would be an attractive model that may meet the enormous demand for the increasing number of elderly inpatients.

Initial enthusiasm for geriatric consultation services had merit. A report out of Halifax, Nova Scotia, Canada, in 1987 by Hogan and colleagues[24] was promising. In 113 patients ages 75 years and older followed for 1 year, the intervention group had greater improvement in mental status, were receiving fewer medications at discharge, and had lower short-term death rates. In 1989, McVey and colleagues[25] published a report from the Veterans Administration Medical Center of North Carolina that showed approximately two-thirds of patients admitted had some degree of functional disability and that geriatric consultative services had a positive impact on the activities of daily living. Sporadic reports continued through the 1990s. Doubt was cast, however, with a meta-analysis in 1993 by Stuck and colleagues[26] reporting no convincing evidence of improvement in clinical or administrative outcomes from geriatric consultation services. A subsequent meta-analysis in 2013 by Deschodt and colleagues[27] did show favorable outcomes in 6-month and 8-month mortality rates (relative risk [RR] 0.66%; 95% CI, 0.52–0.85, and RR 0.51; 95% CI, 0.31–0.85, respectively) but failed to show any significant difference in hospital length of stay, functional status, or readmission rates.

Overall, it remains skeptical that geriatric consultative services alone significantly improve the outcomes of elderly patients in the acute care setting.

GERIATRIC WARDS

Old age is no place for sissies

—Bette Davis

According to published data from the American Hospital Association, fewer than half the hospitals that provide care for the elderly have geriatric wards or offer comprehensive geriatric assessment.[28] Geriatric wards are generally termed, GEM units or acute care of elders (ACE) units. ACE units may focus more specifically on the acute care issues of the patient versus GEM units, which may refer to the longer-term rehabilitation setting. There is no standard that defines a GEM/ACE unit but typically this should entail a discrete ward specifically for the acute care of patients 60 years and older with a multidisciplinary care team dedicated to the care of the elderly. An ACE team typically includes a unit coordinator, geriatrician, pharmacists, physical and occupational therapists, nurses, dietician, and social worker.[29] Functionally, the ward may include improved lighting over that of standard fluorescence, flooring that reduces the risk of fall injury, and devices that optimize orientation or other processes to maintain sleep-wake cycles to reduce delirium.[28]

An exciting 1984 randomized clinical trial of geriatric unit effectiveness cited a 50% reduction in mortality (23.8% vs 48.3%; $P<.005$) and a 50% decrease in the number of patients discharged to a nursing home (12.5% vs 30%; $P<.05$).[30] Additionally, they found that patients in the geriatric ward were more likely to have improvements in functional status, require fewer acute-care hospital days, and face few acute-care hospital readmissions.

Landefeld and colleagues[31] performed a randomized trial of 1794 patients ages 70 and older admitted to an ACE unit versus those admitted to general medical care (GMC). Only 14% of the ACE group patients were discharged to long-term care facilities versus 22% of the GMC group. Additionally a greater proportion of the ACE unit patients reported improvement in activities of daily living (34% vs 24%).

Flood and colleagues[32] showed an ACE unit "significantly reduces variable direct costs and 30-day readmission rates for patients 70 years or older." This translated into approximately $148,400 for every 400 patients admitted to an ACE unit.

A meta-analysis of 28 controlled trials published in *The Lancet* showed the combined odds ratio for a geriatric ward patient to be discharged home to be 1.68 (95% CI, 1.17–2.41). The geriatric ward patients also had a reduction in 6-month mortality with a combined odds ratio of 0.65 (95% CI, 0.46–0.9).[26]

Not all researchers agree on the positive effects of ACE units. A randomized study of outcomes published by Harris and colleagues[33] in 1991 did not find significant differences in outcomes between geriatric units versus general medical units as it related to length of stay, in hospital mortality, or 12-month mortality. In their opinion, admission to geriatric wards based solely on age alone was "medically inappropriate and cost-inefficient."

GERIATRIC MULTIDISCIPLINARY TEAMS

One's destination is never a place, but a new way of looking at things.
—Henry Miller

As health care expenditures continue to rise, acute care hospitals are under pressure to optimize the delivery of care while at the same time maintaining or improving the quality of care. Dedicating a set number of beds (unit) for a specialized purpose logically requires fixed resources, which may translate into fixed assets that have the potential to go underutilized. Thus, it stands to reason that acute care hospitals may prefer maximum flexibility to meet the ebbs and flows of varying demands.

For instance, Mount Sinai Hospital chose to disband their ACE unit in favor of a mobile acute care for elders (MACE) model. The "MACE service team consisted of an attending geriatrician-hospitalist, geriatric medicine fellow, social worker, and a clinical nurse specialist."[29] Hung and colleagues[29] studied the impact of MACE compared with general medical service care for patients ages 75 and older. In this prospective matched cohort of 173 patient pairs, the MACE group had 9.5 adverse events versus 17.06 for the general medical service (adjusted odds ratio 0.11; 95% CI, 0.01–0.88; $P = .04$), shorter hospital stays (0.8 days; 95% CI, 0.8–0.9; $P = .001$), and decreased 30-day readmission rate (odds ratio 0.91; 95% CI, 0.39–2.10; $P = .83$).

Mangram and colleagues[6] studied the geriatric team model in 673 trauma patients, 60 years and older. Although the investigators described admission to "a unit," the model was operationally an interdisciplinary team focused on the needs of the elderly trauma patient. In their "1-year experience," patients experienced decreased time in the emergency department, hospital length of stay, ICU length of stay, and mortality compared with their historical matched controls.

Grund and colleagues[34] evaluated patients over 75 years old with hip and pelvic ring fractures admitted to a geriatric trauma team (GTT) compared with a historical group. The GTT consisted of a comanagement model with a geriatrician and trauma surgeon. They found a reduction in ICU admissions (13.7% vs 20.7%; 95% CI, 9.3%–18.5%; $P = .057$). There was a trend toward decreased mortality (6.5% vs 9.5%; $P = .278$) and decreased ICU length of stay (48 hours vs 53 hours; $P = .973$). There was a statistical increase in overall length of stay for the GTT group (16.9 days vs 13.7 days; $P = .001$). In their subgroup analysis of patients 64 years to 75 years of age, they did not find any comparable trends.

Finally, in a Cochrane database meta-analysis for surgical patients, 8 studies were reviewed; 6 of 8 studies consisted of patients treated for hip fractures and 2 studies involved patients treated for cancer. Overall, they found that patients undergoing a comprehensive geriatric assessment (a process that includes evaluation and care by an interdisciplinary team) "were less likely to die and more likely to return home" than their traditional care counterparts.[35]

SUMMARY

In the acute care surgery/trauma setting, attention to the unique issues of the elderly patient have not been at the forefront of daily practice. Trauma in particular has traditionally been perceived as a young person's disease. For decades, and still today, trauma is the number 1 cause of death for people ages 1 to 44. A very sharp increase, however, in the number of elderly trauma patients and acute care surgery patients is being seen. With this clear increase, a paradigm shift is needed in how surgical and trauma care is delivered.

The field of trauma in particular is undergoing significant changes as it relates to the mechanism of injury for patients ages 60 years and older. Historically, the most common mechanisms of injury for admission after injury were motor vehicle collision, motorcycle collision, gunshot wound, and stab wound. For the past 15 years, there has been a shift to falls as the most frequent reason for admission, especially for the elderly. The level of the fall includes from ground level, ladders, and roofs as well as falls while walking, running, skiing, and hiking. The spectrum of injuries associated with falls in the geriatric population is vast (hip fractures, traumatic brain injuries, spine fractures, intra-abdominal injuries, and more). It is not the injury per se that challenges the surgeon but rather the compounding effect of lowered physiologic reserve, comorbidities, and polypharmacy in the elderly patients.

This article addressed multiple models as they relate to the care of the geriatric surgical patient, whether orthopedic surgery, trauma surgery, acute care surgery, or any other. In the field of medicine, it has been proven that a multidisciplinary approach to the care of the critically ill is best. It seems from the review in this article that a service or team model is associated with improved outcomes when aided by a comprehensive geriatric assessment and management.

Surgeons are simply not trained in geriatric medicine. Out of necessity, they are increasing their understanding of the myriad adverse physiologic and behavioral processes associated with aging. A consultative model that uses the expertise of a geriatrician can be helpful, with expertise of management of hypertension, arrhythmias, diabetes, and chronic obstructive pulmonary disease along with advanced training in the psychosocial issues of the elderly. However, there still is not sufficient evidence to state that the standard of care requires that a geriatrician be consulted for all elderly patient admissions. Notwithstanding, there simply are not enough trained geriatricians to take on the Sisyphean task found today.

The multidisciplinary approach is discussed multiple times in this article. This approach can be geographically defined as geriatric units or be more fluidic in approach. The multidisciplinary model seems associated with improved outcomes.

In particular, the authors' results with a surgeon-led, G60 trauma model are discussed, referencing that people are living more active lives and living longer, with current life expectancy at 78 years compared with the 1900s when life expectancy was 50 years. So there may be a transition from caring for the frail to the active elder. Nevertheless, a team approach is the model of choice that is recommended to become the standard of care. Further studies regarding surgical and trauma care for the elderly should be ongoing. In closing, the boom of elderly trauma patients is not coming... It is already here.

REFERENCES

1. Committee on the Future Health Care Workforce for Older Americans, Board on Health Care Services. Retooling for an aging America: building the health care workforce. 1st edition. Washington, DC: National Academies Press; 2008.

2. Ritchie C, Andersen R, Eng J, et al. Implementation of an interdisciplinary, team-based complex care support health care model at an academic medical center: impact on health care utilization and quality of life. PLoS One 2016;11(2). https://doi.org/10.1371/journal.pone.0148096.

3. Joyce MF, Gupta A, Azocar RJ. Acute trauma and multiple injuries in the elderly population. Curr Opin Anaesthesiol 2015;28(2):145–50.

4. Schwab CW, Kauder DR. Trauma in the geriatric patient. Arch Surg 1992;127(6):701–6.

5. Jacobs DG. Special considerations in geriatric injury. Curr Opin Crit Care 2003;9(6):535–9.

6. Mangram AJ, Mitchell CD, Shifflette VK, et al. Geriatric trauma service: a one-year experience. J Trauma Acute Care Surg 2012;72(1):119–22.

7. Scalea TM, Simon HM, Duncan AO, et al. Geriatric blunt multiple trauma: improved survival with early invasive monitoring. J Trauma 1990;30(2):129–34 [discussion: 134–6].

8. Demetriades D, Karaiskakis M, Velmahos G, et al. Effect on outcome of early intensive management of geriatric trauma patients. Br J Surg 2002;89(10):1319–22.

9. McKinley BA, Marvin RG, Cocanour CS, et al. Blunt trauma resuscitation: the old can respond. Arch Surg 2000;135(6):688–93 [discussion: 694–5].

10. McMahon DJ, Schwab CW, Kauder D. Comorbidity and the elderly trauma patient. World J Surg 1996;20(8):1113–9 [discussion: 1119–20].

11. Piccirillo JF, Vlahiotis A, Barrett LB, et al. The changing prevalence of comorbidity across the age spectrum. Crit Rev Oncol Hematol 2008;67(2):124–32.

12. Joseph B, Pandit V, Sadoun M, et al. Frailty in surgery. J Trauma Acute Care Surg 2014;76(4):1151–6.

13. Mangram A, Corneille M, Moyer M, et al. Pre-injury VES-13 score at admission predicts discharge disposition for geriatric trauma patients. Ann Gerontol Geriatr Res 2014;1(2):1–4.

14. Dzandu JK, Mangram AJ, Corneille MG, et al. Pre-injury vulnerable elders survey (VES-13) score facilitates initiation of hospital discharge planning for older trauma patients on admission. J Am Coll Surg 2014;219(4):e52.

15. Maxwell CA, Mion LC, Mukherjee K, et al. Preinjury physical frailty and cognitive impairment among geriatric trauma patients determine postinjury functional recovery and survival. J Trauma Acute Care Surg 2016;80(2):195–203.

16. Maxwell CA, Dietrich MS, Minnick AF, et al. Preinjury physical function and frailty in injured older adults: self- versus proxy responses. J Am Geriatr Soc 2015;63(7):1443–7.

17. Joseph B, Pandit V, Zangbar B, et al. Superiority of frailty over age in predicting outcomes among geriatric trauma patients: a prospective analysis. JAMA Surg 2014;149(8):766–72.

18. Joseph B, Pandit V, Rhee P, et al. Predicting hospital discharge disposition in geriatric trauma patients: is frailty the answer? J Trauma Acute Care Surg 2014;76(1):196–200.

19. St-Louis E, Sudarshan M, Al-Habboubi M, et al. The outcomes of the elderly in acute care general surgery. Eur J Trauma Emerg Surg 2016;42(1):107–13.

20. Joseph B, Zangbar B, Pandit V, et al. Emergency general surgery in the elderly: too old or too frail? J Am Coll Surg 2016;222(5):805–13.

21. Farhat JS, Velanovich V, Falvo AJ, et al. Are the frail destined to fail? Frailty index as predictor of surgical morbidity and mortality in the elderly. J Trauma Acute Care Surg 2012;72(6):1526–30 [discussion: 1530–1].

22. Pioli G, Giusti A, Barone A. Orthogeriatric care for the elderly with hip fractures: where are we? Aging Clin Exp Res 2008;20(2):113–22.
23. Rubenstein LZ, Stuck AE, Siu AL, et al. Impacts of geriatric evaluation and management programs on defined outcomes: overview of the evidence. J Am Geriatr Soc 1991;39(9 Pt 2):8S–16S [discussion: 17S–18S].
24. Hogan DB, Fox RA, Badley BW, et al. Effect of a geriatric consultation service on management of patients in an acute care hospital. CMAJ 1987;136(7):713–7.
25. McVey LJ, Becker PM, Saltz CC, et al. Effect of a geriatric consultation team on functional status of elderly hospitalized patients. Ann Intern Med 1989;110(1):79–84.
26. Stuck AE, Siu AL, Wieland GD, et al. Comprehensive geriatric assessment: a meta-analysis of controlled trials. Lancet 1993;342(8878):1032–6.
27. Deschodt M, Flamaing J, Haentjens P, et al. Impact of geriatric consultation teams on clinical outcome in acute hospitals: a systematic review and meta-analysis. BMC Med 2013;11(1). https://doi.org/10.1186/1741-7015-11-48.
28. Agency for Healthcare Research and Quality. Chapter 30. Geriatric evaluation and management units for hospitalized patients. Available at: https://archive.ahrq.gov/clinic/ptsafety/chap30.htm. Accessed March 26, 2018.
29. Hung WW, Ross JS, Farber J, et al. Evaluation of a mobile acute care for the elderly service. JAMA Intern Med 2013;173(11):990–6.
30. Rubenstein LZ, Josephson KR, Wieland GD, et al. Effectiveness of a geriatric evaluation unit. A randomized clinical trial. N Engl J Med 1984;311(26):1664–70.
31. Landefeld CS, Palmer RM, Kresevic DM, et al. A randomized trial of care in a hospital medical unit especially designed to improve the functional outcomes of acutely ill older patients. N Engl J Med 1995;332(20):1338–44.
32. Flood KL, Maclennan PA, McGrew D, et al. Effects of an acute care for elders unit on costs and 30-day readmissions. JAMA Intern Med 2013;173(11):981–7.
33. Harris RD, Henschke PJ, Popplewell PY, et al. A randomised study of outcomes in a defined group of acutely ill elderly patients managed in a geriatric assessment unit or a general medical unit. Aust N Z J Med 1991;21(2):230–4.
34. Grund S, Roos M, Duchene W, et al. Treatment in a center for geriatric traumatology. Dtsch Arztebl Int 2015;112(7):113–9.
35. Eamer G, Taheri A, Chen SS, et al. Comprehensive geriatric assessment for older people admitted to a surgical service. Cochrane Database Syst Rev 2018;(1):CD012485.

Palliative Care and Geriatric Surgery

Jessica H. Ballou, MD, MPH, Karen J. Brasel, MD, MPH*

KEYWORDS

- Geriatric surgery • Palliative care • Palliative surgery • Goals of care
- Advance directives

KEY POINTS

- Surgical patients are at high risk of having unmet palliative care needs and generally have low referral rates to specialty palliative care services.
- A large proportion of elderly surgical patients lack decision-making capacity near the end of life.
- Palliative surgical procedures can be considered for symptom relief in certain incurable diseases, even in patients with do-not-resuscitate orders.

INTRODUCTION

Historically, advanced age alone was a contraindication to operative intervention.[1] Today, however, medical advances in technique and technology allow both cardiac and noncardiac operations to be safely performed in elderly patients.[2–4] Although resource capabilities may dictate what can be done for geriatric patients, determining what should be done is far more difficult. A growing body of literature reveals that seniors often describe outcomes—especially maintaining quality of life or independence—as a priority over life-prolonging procedures.[5–8] When asked about their end-of-life wishes, many older persons express the desire to die at home in control of their health care decisions.[9,10]

Despite these preferences, a vast majority of Americans die in hospitals (53%) or nursing homes (24%),[9] and approximately a third of Medicare decedents undergo a surgical procedure or are admitted to the ICU in their last year of life.[11–13] This discrepancy between desired outcomes and reality underscores the growing emphasis on palliative care in geriatric surgical patients by the American College of Surgery, National Academy of Medicine, and other health care agencies.[14,15]

Disclosure Statement: The authors have nothing to disclose.
Department of Surgery, Oregon Health & Science University, 3181 Southwest Sam Jackson Park Road, Portland, OR 97239, USA
* Corresponding author.
E-mail address: brasel@ohsu.edu

Clin Geriatr Med 35 (2019) 35–44
https://doi.org/10.1016/j.cger.2018.08.004
0749-0690/19/© 2018 Elsevier Inc. All rights reserved.
geriatric.theclinics.com

DEFINING PALLIATIVE CARE

Palliative care refers to multidisciplinary interventions to relieve pain and other symptoms associated with advanced illness in an effort to enhance quality of life for patients and their families.[15] As a specialty, palliative care has been shown to enhance quality of life[16] while at times improving survival,[17] limiting in-hospital deaths,[18] and reducing costs mainly by reducing length of stay.[19–21]

The focus on symptom relief need not be limited to the end of life. Palliative care may span an entire course of treatment of a serious illness and be offered by a range of providers in a variety of settings, including hospitals, nursing homes, outpatient clinics, and hospice.[15] **Box 1** provides definitions of the diverse applications of palliative care.

IDENTIFYING THOSE IN GREATEST NEED OF PALLIATIVE CARE

Palliative care consultations are less common in surgical patients than in patients with chronic medical illnesses and are often delayed until patients are within days of death.[24,25] Although all patients benefit from basic palliative care, it is essential to identify those at greatest need of specialized palliative care because palliative care specialists cannot and should not manage all seriously ill patients.[23] The Center to Advance Palliative Care recommends a palliative care assessment be completed on hospital admission.[23] The palliative care assessment can be done by any member of the treatment team and does not require specialized palliative training.

Depending on the complexity of the responses and the resources of the primary treatment team, answers to these questions may or may not result in a specialist

---

Box 1
Palliative care definitions

Palliative care: care that provides relief from pain and other symptoms, supports quality of life, and is focused on patients with serious advanced illness and their families.

Basic palliative care: palliative care that is delivered by health care professionals, such as primary care clinicians; physicians who are disease-oriented specialists (such as oncologists and cardiologists); and nurses, social workers, pharmacists, chaplains, and others who care for this population but are not certified in palliative care.

Specialty palliative care: palliative care that is delivered by health care professionals who are palliative care specialists, such as physicians who are board certified in this specialty; palliative-certified nurses; and palliative care–certified social workers, pharmacists, and chaplains.

End-of-life care: processes of addressing the medical, social, emotional, and spiritual needs of people who are nearing the end of life. It may include a range of medical and social services, including disease-specific interventions as well as palliative and hospice care for those with advanced serious conditions who are near the end of life.

Hospice: an interdisciplinary approach to deliver medical, nursing, social, psychological, emotional, and spiritual services through a collaboration of professionals and other caregivers, with the goal of making terminally ill persons (life expectancy typically ≤ 6 months) as physically and emotionally comfortable as possible.[22]

Goals of care: physical, social, spiritual, or other patient-centered goals that arise after an informed discussion of the current disease(s), prognosis, and treatment options.[23]

Adapted from Institute of Medicine. 2015. Dying in America: Improving Quality and Honoring Individual Preferences Near the End of Life. Washington, DC: The National Academies Press. https://doi.org/10.17226/18748.

palliative care referral. There are certain clinical criteria, however, that should trigger consideration of specialist palliative care consultation.[23] These include

- The surprise question: You would not be surprised if the patient died within 12 months.
- Frequent admissions, in particular to the ICU.[26]
- Admission prompted by challenging physical or psychological symptoms
- Complex care requirements
- Decline in function, feeding intolerance, or failure to thrive
- ICU length of stay greater than or equal to 7 days

There is a relative dearth of studies evaluating the impact of palliative care triggers in surgical ICUs compared with medical ICUs. The medical ICU triggers, however, are associated with shorter ICU and hospital length of stay and more proactive discussions of goals of care without increased mortality.[26,27] Nonetheless, the American College of Surgeons Surgical Palliative Care Task Force has identified specific conditions for surgical patients to consider involving palliative care specialists[27]:

- Family request
- Family disagreement with team, advance directive or each other (lasting >4 days)
- Glasgow Outcome Scale score 3 (ie, persistent vegetative state)
- Futility considered or declared by medical team
- Death expected during same surgical ICU stay
- A diagnosis with median survival less than 6 months
- Carcinomatosis or unresectable malignancy
- Presence of an advanced directive authorizing withdrawal of (life-sustaining measures)
- Glasgow Coma Scale score less than 8 for greater than 1 week in a patient greater than 55 years old
- Multisystem organ failure

Each institution faces its own limitations with regard to its resources for managing palliative care needs and referrals. Furthermore, these assessments were developed for hospitalized patients or those already stressed by acute illness. Although hospitalized elderly patients are likely to need palliative interventions, the groundwork for preemptive symptom relief and goals of care can ideally be done prior to needing hospitalization.

CLINICAL VIGNETTE

Mr. B is a 70-year-old man with diabetes, chronic obstructive pulmonary disease, and coronary artery disease who presents for a wellness visit. He lives alone and comes in at the encouragement of his adult children after not seeking care in the 5 years since his wife's death. He reports that he has mild shortness of breath with exertion but otherwise has no complaints. With his history of smoking, he is referred for a screening abdominal ultrasound that reveals a 6-cm abdominal aortic aneurysm. You inform him that his aneurysm meets criteria for operative repair and he asks what should be done.

PALLIATIVE CARE PLANNING IN THE ELECTIVE SETTING
Managing Trade-offs

It would be both feasible and historically accurate for the physician to make a referral to a surgeon and for Mr. B to move forward with a procedure on the implicit trust that the referral meant surgery was in his best interest. Mr. B may have perceived no other options.[28] Recordings of preoperative encounters for elderly patients undergoing high-risk procedures reveal that although surgeons do discuss the potential for serious complications, these conversations rarely include discussions of prolonged life-supporting treatments or what complications would be unacceptable to the patient.[29]

Focus groups of elderly individuals reveal 3 major influences on treatment preferences: treatment burden, treatment outcome, and the likelihood of the outcome.[7] What constitutes an acceptable burden, outcome, or likelihood of outcome varies between patients and can change for individual patients over time.[30] Ultimately, what is needed is a more holistic version of the informed consent to include a detailed discussion of patient preferences and goals to allow for shared decision making between physician and patient.

Shared Decision Making and Eliciting Goals of Care

To elicit a patient's goals of care and identify the factors that contribute to quality of life, the American College of Critical Care Medicine Ethics Committee and the American Thoracic Society, among others, emphasize the importance of shared decision making. Shared decision making refers to the "collaborative process that allows patients, or their surrogates, and clinicians to make healthcare decisions together, taking into account the best scientific evidence available, as well as the patient's values, goals, and preferences."[31] Although typically used to in critical care settings, the 2 main elements of shared decision making—information exchange, deliberation, and making a treatment decision—can be used by providers in a variety of settings.[31]

Communication aids for elective surgery have been developed to assist with information exchange and decision making in high-risk operations. A question prompt list (QPL) was developed after recorded sessions between patients and providers as well as patients and family members with personal experience of having been through a high-risk surgery.[32] Rather than discuss the logistics of the procedure (eg, "Will there be sutures or staples?"), the QPL encourages discussions in three broad areas[32]:

- Should I have surgery?
- What should I expect if everything goes well?
- What happens if things go wrong?

Although further research is needed to determine the extent to which tools, such as the QPL, have an impact on treatment decisions and reduce postoperative conflicts, these questions shift the focus from technical details to aligning patient goals with possible procedure outcomes.

PALLIATIVE CARE IN THE EMERGENT SETTING

While awaiting the appointment to discuss surgical repair of his aneurysm, Mr. B experiences acute-onset severe lower back pain. He is brought to the emergency department by ambulance and a rapid assessment reveals that the aneurysm has ruptured. He is awake but uncomfortable and appears distressed. He has no family members present but he says his oldest daughter is on her way.

On any given day, up to a quarter of all emergency hospital admissions are for general surgical conditions.[33] Although outcomes for elective operations in geriatric patients can rival younger patients, there is strong evidence of higher morbidity and mortality for geriatric patients undergoing emergency surgery for illness or trauma.[34–36] Although these findings may be due to frailty more than absolute age,[37] a review of approximately 40,000 patients who underwent an emergency laparotomy showed that American Society of Anesthesiologists (ASA) classification, functional status, sepsis, and age were significantly associated with mortality.[38] In this study, patients older than 90 years of age with an ASA class V, septic shock, dependent functional status, and abnormal white blood cell count have a less than 10% probability of survival.[38] Even in cases of patients surviving their acute illness, emergency procedures in the elderly are associated with high complication rates and loss of function.[4] In a study of octogenarians undergoing open type A aortic aneurysm repair, 40% of patients returned home with "satisfactory autonomy" but every patient had a decrease in performance status postoperatively.[39]

From the surgeon's perspective, the decision regarding whether to proceed with surgery is heavily influenced by past experiences. In their focus group of surgeons discussing a hypothetical high-risk procedure on an elderly patient, Nabozny and colleagues[5] found that "some surgeons believed the likelihood of a good outcome was so small and the burdens of treatment were so high, that they would not offer surgery to the patients. Others reported that they would offer and perform surgery if the patient and/or family insisted, but they would frame the decision-making conversation in a way that would bias the choice against surgery." They went on to further describe the "clinical momentum" wherein some surgeons felt a need to conform to a surgical treatment plan that began with the referring physician.[5]

Difficult Conversations Between Strangers

Emergency situations leave providers and patients little time for introductions and discussions of goals of care or end-of-life preferences. In severe cases, patients and physicians may believe they are being forced to make a choice between palliative care or surgery. Despite the generally agreed-on goal of maximizing quality of life and independence, this dichotomization results in 1 of 2 perspectives: (1) that the choice being made is whether to live (surgery) or die (palliative care) or (2) that death is the likely outcome of either path and the choice being made is how to die.[5] Nabozny and colleagues[5] found that seniors who viewed the choice as live versus die also had the unfounded belief that surgery could be attempted and easily abandoned if unsuccessful and that death, if it occurred, would be painless in the operating room. These beliefs were present regardless of the surgeon's explicit statement that postoperative deaths usually follow a prolonged course in the ICU.

Both the patient and the physician face the challenge of incomplete information and biases based on their past experiences. One method of information exchange in such situations is called best case/worst case and involves a visual representation of the best, worst, and most likely outcomes for patients facing the decision of whether or not to proceed with surgery.[40]

The best case/worst case communication tool allows both physician and patient to visualize the spectrum of possible outcomes with their associated probabilities based on the physician's experience.[40] The patient can then get an idea of the treatment burdens, treatment outcomes, and the likelihood of the outcomes as they pertain to their individual circumstances.

WHEN A PATIENT CANNOT COMMUNICATE

Although it would be ideal for patients to fully participate in their own medical decisions, a substantial proportion of hospitalized elderly patients lack the capacity to make their own medical decisions due to either acute or chronic illness.[41,42] As a result, physicians must rely on the patient's previously stated wishes (advance directives) or a surrogate decision maker.

Advance Directives

Although advance directives are intended to guide patient treatments and relieve families or surrogates from the burden of making treatment decisions, their real-world application in geriatric patients undergoing high-risk operations is unclear.[43,44] Studies comparing patient preferences to care received demonstrate racial, cultural, geographic, and religious discrepancies regarding who completes advance directives and whether or not they are followed.[41,45–47] A 2012 survey of vascular surgeons, cardiac surgeons, and neurosurgeons who perform high-risk operations in elderly patients found that only 60% report always or sometimes discussing advance directives with patients.[48] These surgeons also noted that the although the principal determinants of whether to proceed with surgery were postoperative quality of life and comorbidities, the presence of an existing do-not-resuscitate (DNR) order was a factor when declining an operation.[48]

Surrogates and the Unbefriended or Unrepresented Patient

When a patient is unable to communicate and an advance directive is unclear or unavailable, treatment decisions fall to the patient's surrogate. This, unfortunately, represents a substantial proportion of elderly patients. Using the Health and Retirement Study data, Silveira and colleagues[41] found that 70% of decedents over age 60 who required medical decisions at the end of life lacked capacity and one-third lacked an advanced directive. All 50 states have some form of delineation for the lineage of surrogacy but who may make the decisions and the order of priority varies from state to state.[49]

Patients with no surrogate—the unbefriended or unrepresented patients—present significant ethical challenges when no advance directive is available. Although hospitals and legal systems may have methods to identifies proxies for a patient, these can be cumbersome or impractical in certain circumstances.[50] As a result, clinicians may be put in a position to exercise substituted judgment on behalf of unrepresented patients while efforts to find a surrogate take place.[50,51] Early recognition of unrepresented patients and discussions of advance directives are essential because these patients are at particularly high risk of not having their care wishes met, particularly in emergencies because the default is to treat unless the circumstances are deemed futile.[52]

SURGICAL PALLIATION

Surgical palliation refers to procedures for patients with incurable disease that are intended to "relieve symptoms, minimize patient distress, and improve quality of life" and are typically performed for relief from obstruction, bleeding, perforation, or intractable pain.[53] Any procedure that relieves symptoms may be considered palliative, and the presence of an advance directive specifying comfort care or DNR order does not negate the possibility of surgery.[54] Prior to chemotherapy regimens and comprehensive medical therapies, many of the procedures that are considered life-prolonging originated as palliative procedures to relieve pain and discomfort. Radical mastectomy, for example, was described by Halsted to reduce the pain associated from advanced breast cancer while coronary artery bypass grafting was performed to reduce angina.[53,55]

Although these procedures may be associated with brief periods of discomfort or hospitalizations, many patients find that they improve or at least do not diminish quality of life.[56] Given the incurable nature of the underlying conditions, outcomes for palliative surgeries are measured by relief of the targeted symptoms rather than standard surgical measures, such as 30-day mortality.[57] In all cases, it is important to take into consideration individual level of frailty, symptoms, likelihood of success and durability of the procedure, availability and efficacy of nonsurgical management, and the patient's quality and expectancy of life.[58]

SUMMARY

At its core, palliative care refers to the treatment of the person rather than the disease. Although specialty palliative care is now available at most major medical centers, the majority of palliative care for geriatric surgical patients falls to community physicians and surgeons. Fortunately, effective discussions of treatment outcomes, burdens, and likelihood of outcomes do not require specialty training in palliative care. Through united, multidisciplinary efforts to identify the factors associated with quality, not just quantity, of life for patients, meeting the palliative care needs of a growing geriatric population can be started.

REFERENCES

1. Neuman MD, Bosk CL. The redefinition of aging in American surgery. Milbank Q 2013;91(2):288–315.
2. Gervasi R, Orlando G, Lerose MA, et al. Thyroid surgery in geriatric patients: a literature review. BMC Surg 2012;12(Suppl 1):S16.
3. Pallati PK, Gupta PK, Bichala S, et al. Short-term outcomes of inguinal hernia repair in octogenarians and nonagenarians. Hernia 2013;17(6):723–7.
4. Farina-Castro R, Roque-Castellano C, Marchena-Gomez J, et al. Five-year survival after surgery in nonagenarian patients. Geriatr Gerontol Int 2017;17(12): 2389–95.
5. Nabozny MJ, Kruser JM, Steffens NM, et al. Constructing high-stakes surgical decisions: it's better to die trying. Ann Surg 2016;263(1):64–70.
6. Fried TR, Bradley EH, Towle VR, et al. Understanding the treatment preferences of seriously ill patients. N Engl J Med 2002;346(14):1061–6.
7. Fried TR, Bradley EH. What matters to seriously ill older persons making end-of-life treatment decisions?: A qualitative study. J Palliat Med 2003;6(2):237–44.
8. Rosenfeld KE, Wenger NS, Kagawa-Singer M. End-of-life decision making: a qualitative study of elderly individuals. J Gen Intern Med 2000;15(9):620–5.
9. Gruneir A, Mor V, Weitzen S, et al. Where people die: a multilevel approach to understanding influences on site of death in America. Med Care Res Rev 2007; 64(4):351–78.
10. Tang ST. When death is imminent: where terminally ill patients with cancer prefer to die and why. Cancer Nurs 2003;26(3):245–51.
11. Kwok AC, Semel ME, Lipsitz SR, et al. The intensity and variation of surgical care at the end of life: a retrospective cohort study. Lancet 2011;378(9800):1408–13.
12. Teno JM, Gozalo PL, Bynum JP, et al. Change in end-of-life care for medicare beneficiaries: site of death, place of care, and health care transitions in 2000, 2005, and 2009. JAMA 2013;309(5):470–7.
13. Angus DC, Barnato AE, Linde-Zwirble WT, et al. Use of intensive care at the end of life in the United States: an epidemiologic study. Crit Care Med 2004;32(3): 638–43.
14. Mosenthal AC. Palliative care in the surgical ICU. Surg Clin North Am 2005;85(2): 303–13.
15. National Academy of Medicine. Dying in America: improving quality and honoring individual preferences near the end of life. Washington, DC: National Academies Press; 2015.

16. Casarett D, Johnson M, Smith D, et al. The optimal delivery of palliative care: a national comparison of the outcomes of consultation teams vs inpatient units. Arch Intern Med 2011;171(7):649–55.

17. Temel JS, Greer JA, Muzikansky A, et al. Early palliative care for patients with metastatic non-small-cell lung cancer. N Engl J Med 2010;363(8):733–42.

18. Yoo JW, Nakagawa S, Kim S. Integrative palliative care, advance directives, and hospital outcomes of critically ill older adults. Am J Hosp Palliat Care 2012;29(8): 655–62.

19. May P, Garrido MM, Cassel JB, et al. Cost analysis of a prospective multi-site cohort study of palliative care consultation teams for adults with advanced cancer: where do cost-savings come from? Palliat Med 2017;31(4):378–86.

20. Ciemins EL, Blum L, Nunley M, et al. The economic and clinical impact of an inpatient palliative care consultation service: a multifaceted approach. J Palliat Med 2007;10(6):1347–55.

21. May P, Normand C, Morrison RS. Economic impact of hospital inpatient palliative care consultation: review of current evidence and directions for future research. J Palliat Med 2014;17(9):1054–63.

22. Medicare Program; FY 2018 hospice wage index and payment rate update and hospice quality reporting requirements. In: services DoHAHSCfMaM, editor. vol. 82. Washington DC: 2017. Available at: http://www.nhpco.org/sites/default/files/public/regulatory/FY2017_Final-Hospice-Wage-Index-Rule_080116.pdf. Accessed September 19, 2018.

23. Weissman DE, Meier DE. Identifying patients in need of a palliative care assessment in the hospital setting: a consensus report from the Center to Advance Palliative Care. J Palliat Med 2011;14(1):17–23.

24. Lilley EJ, Cooper Z, Schwarze ML, et al. Palliative care in surgery: defining the research priorities. Ann Surg 2018;267(1):66–72.

25. Rivet EB, Ferrada P, Albrecht T, et al. Characteristics of palliative care consultation at an academic level one trauma center. Am J Surg 2017;214(4):657–60.

26. Finkelstein M, Goldstein NE, Horton JR, et al. Developing triggers for the surgical intensive care unit for palliative care integration. J Crit Care 2016;35:7–11.

27. Bradley CT, Brasel KJ. Developing guidelines that identify patients who would benefit from palliative care services in the surgical intensive care unit. Crit Care Med 2009;37(3):946–50.

28. Schwarze ML, Brasel KJ, Mosenthal AC. Beyond 30-day mortality: aligning surgical quality with outcomes that patients value. JAMA Surg 2014;149(7):631–2.

29. Pecanac KE, Kehler JM, Brasel KJ, et al. It's big surgery: preoperative expressions of risk, responsibility, and commitment to treatment after high-risk operations. Ann Surg 2014;259(3):458–63.

30. Fried TR, Van Ness PH, Byers AL, et al. Changes in preferences for life-sustaining treatment among older persons with advanced illness. J Gen Intern Med 2007; 22(4):495–501.

31. Kon AA, Davidson JE, Morrison W, et al. Shared decision making in ICUs: an American College of critical care medicine and American Thoracic Society policy statement. Crit Care Med 2016;44(1):188–201.

32. Steffens NM, Tucholka JL, Nabozny MJ, et al. Engaging patients, health care professionals, and community members to improve preoperative decision making for older adults facing high-risk surgery. JAMA Surg 2016;151(10):938–45.

33. Desserud KF, Veen T, Soreide K. Emergency general surgery in the geriatric patient. Br J Surg 2016;103(2):e52–61.

34. Hashmi A, Ibrahim-Zada I, Rhee P, et al. Predictors of mortality in geriatric trauma patients: a systematic review and meta-analysis. J Trauma Acute Care Surg 2014; 76(3):894–901.

35. Adams SD, Holcomb JB. Geriatric trauma. Curr Opin Crit Care 2015;21(6):520–6.

36. Zafar SN, Obirieze A, Schneider EB, et al. Outcomes of trauma care at centers treating a higher proportion of older patients: the case for geriatric trauma centers. J Trauma Acute Care Surg 2015;78(4):852–9.

37. Joseph B, Zangbar B, Pandit V, et al. Emergency general surgery in the elderly: too old or too frail? J Am Coll Surg 2016;222(5):805–13.

38. Al-Temimi MH, Griffee M, Enniss TM, et al. When is death inevitable after emergency laparotomy? Analysis of the American College of Surgeons National Surgical Quality Improvement Program database. J Am Coll Surg 2012;215(4):503–11.

39. Vanhuyse F, Maureira P, Laurent N, et al. Surgery for acute type A aortic dissection in octogenarians. J Card Surg 2012;27(1):65–9.

40. Schwarze ML, Kehler JM, Campbell TC. Navigating high risk procedures with more than just a street map. J Palliat Med 2013;16(10):1169–71.

41. Silveira MJ, Kim SY, Langa KM. Advance directives and outcomes of surrogate decision making before death. N Engl J Med 2010;362(13):1211–8.

42. Barnett MD, Williams BR, Tucker RO. Sudden advanced illness: an emerging concept among palliative care and surgical critical care physicians. Am J Hosp Palliat Care 2016;33(4):321–6.

43. Beach MC, Morrison RS. The effect of do-not-resuscitate orders on physician decision-making. J Am Geriatr Soc 2002;50(12):2057–61.

44. Wooster M, Stassi A, Hill J, et al. End-of-life decision-making for patients with geriatric trauma cared for in a trauma intensive care unit. Am J Hosp Palliat Care 2018;35(8):1063–8.

45. Blank RH. End-of-life decision making across cultures. J Law Med Ethics 2011; 39(2):201–14.

46. LoPresti MA, Dement F, Gold HT. End-of-life care for people with cancer from ethnic minority groups: a systematic review. Am J Hosp Palliat Care 2016; 33(3):291–305.

47. Schweda M, Schicktanz S, Raz A, et al. Beyond cultural stereotyping: views on end-of-life decision making among religious and secular persons in the USA, Germany, and Israel. BMC Med Ethics 2017;18(1):13.

48. Redmann AJ, Brasel KJ, Alexander CG, et al. Use of advance directives for high-risk operations: a national survey of surgeons. Ann Surg 2012;255(3): 418–23.

49. DeMartino ES, Dudzinski DM, Doyle CK, et al. Who decides when a patient can't? Statutes on alternate decision makers. N Engl J Med 2017;376(15):1478–82.

50. Pope TM. Making medical decisions for patients without surrogates. N Engl J Med 2013;369(21):1976–8.

51. White DB, Jonsen A, Lo B. Ethical challenge: when clinicians act as surrogates for unrepresented patients. Am J Crit Care 2012;21(3):202–7.

52. Bosslet GT, Pope TM, Rubenfeld GD, et al. An official ATS/AACN/ACCP/ESICM/ SCCM policy statement: responding to requests for potentially inappropriate treatments in intensive care units. Am J Respir Crit Care Med 2015;191(11): 1318–30.

53. Miner TJ. Communication as a core skill of palliative surgical care. Anesthesiol Clin 2012;30(1):47–58.

54. Siracuse JJ, Jones DW, Meltzer EC, et al. Impact of "Do Not Resuscitate" status on the outcome of major vascular surgical procedures. Ann Vasc Surg 2015; 29(7):1339–45.

55. Dunn GP, Milch RA. Introduction and historical background of palliative care: where does the surgeon fit in? J Am Coll Surg 2001;193(3):325–8.

56. Miner TJ. Palliative surgery for advanced cancer: lessons learned in patient selection and outcome assessment. Am J Clin Oncol 2005;28(4):411–4.

57. Lilley EJ, Lindvall C, Lillemoe KD, et al. Measuring processes of care in palliative surgery: a novel approach using natural language processing. Ann Surg 2018; 267(5):823–5.

58. Miner TJ, Cohen J, Charpentier K, et al. The palliative triangle: improved patient selection and outcomes associated with palliative operations. Arch Surg 2011; 146(5):517–22.

Transitions of Care in Geriatric Medicine

Shailvi Gupta, MD, MPH[a], Justin A. Perry, MSW[b], Rosemary Kozar, MD, PhD[c],*

KEYWORDS

- Geriatric trauma • Elderly postoperative • Transitions of care • Discharge destination

KEY POINTS

- Discharge destination after the index hospitalization is a determinant of long-term survival in injured or postoperative elderly patients.
- Many geriatric patients have barriers to successful transitions of care that long predate their acute hospitalization. Rapid assessment and targeted intervention are key to avoiding delays in discharge.
- Prehabilitation prior to elective surgery may be beneficial for the elderly surgical patient to decrease post–acute care facility placement.
- Frequent communication among the interdisciplinary team, including the patient and family along with post–acute care and primary care providers, can reduce readmissions and increase adherence with discharge recommendations.

INTRODUCTION

The elderly population in the United States is predicted to more than double to 80 million by 2050.[1] As the population ages, the elderly are increasingly seeking and requiring medical care, including surgery.[2] Similarly, the number of injured elderly seen in US trauma centers is increasing exponentially.[3] Trauma is the now the seventh leading cause of death in individuals over 65 years of age.[4] Patients who survive their acute injury and/or surgery are faced with a prolonged road to recovery, which includes care beyond acute hospitalization. The transition of care for these elderly patients is paramount to their long-term survival and quality of life and poses complex challenges to health care providers, patients, and their families.

Disclosure: The authors have nothing to disclose.
Funding: There is no associated funding.
[a] Shock Trauma Center, University of Maryland School of Medicine, T1R51, 22 South Greene Street, Baltimore, MD 21201, USA; [b] Department of Care Management, University of Maryland Medical Center, 22 South Greene Street, N1E10A, Baltimore, MD 21201, USA; [c] Shock Trauma Center, University of Maryland School of Medicine, T1R40, 22 South Green Street, Baltimore, MD 21201, USA
* Corresponding author.
E-mail address: rkozar@umm.edu

Clin Geriatr Med 35 (2019) 45–52
https://doi.org/10.1016/j.cger.2018.08.005
0749-0690/19/© 2018 Elsevier Inc. All rights reserved.

IMPORTANCE OF DISCHARGE DESTINATION

Elderly trauma patients are at increased risk for morbidity and mortality after injury in both inpatient and the postdischarge settings.[5] The importance of discharge destination after the index hospitalization is, therefore, increasingly recognized as a determinant of long-term survival in the injured elderly.[6] A large retrospective study found that preexisting comorbid medical conditions increased the odds of complications during the acute hospitalization and also that increasing age, number and types of injuries, injuries due to falls, and lower functional level all predicted discharge to a skilled nursing facility (SNF).[7] Predictors of discharge to an SNF for older trauma patients in Australia included older age, greater injury severity, longer hospital stay, and injury caused by a fall.[8] Beaulieu and colleagues[9] identified early factors predictive of nonhome discharges from a review of 2800 geriatric trauma patients. Independent predictors of disposition to nursing home were female gender, age, intensive care stay, and hospital length of stay. Comorbidities most associated with nonhome disposition were neurologic disorders, coagulopathy, and diabetes mellitus.

After analyzing 1352 geriatric admissions secondary to ground-level falls, Ayoung-Chee and colleagues[10] found 51% of elderly patients were discharged to an SNF, 39% to home, and only 5% to inpatient rehabilitation facilities. As increasing numbers of elderly patients are discharged to SNFs, an increasing number of studies are reporting lower survival for trauma patients discharged to SNFs compared with those discharged to home.[6] Thus, discharge to a SNF is one of the most important independent predictors of poor long-term outcomes for the injured elderly.

Among those older than 65 years and undergoing elective surgery, 45% have ongoing care needs after hospital discharge and require post–acute care services, such as home health care, SNFs, and inpatient rehabilitation.[11,12] Even if functionally independent prior to surgery and without postoperative complications, older surgical patients are also frequently discharged to SNFs.

Hakkarainen and colleagues[13] found that the risk of death at 1 year was highest among patients readmitted to an acute care hospital from the SNF, those remaining in an SNF at 6 months, or those transitioned to assisted living facilities. Furthermore, a significant proportion of patients never returned to home after their admission to an SNF.

In a recent study by Thornblade and colleagues,[14] the investigators reported the effect of nursing ratio and specialty beds in elderly trauma and surgical patients who were discharged to Medicare-certified SNFs. The investigators found that SNFs with fewer beds per nurse had lower mortality, readmissions, and failure to discharge home. Additionally, SNFs with a greater number of specialty beds also had a lower rate of readmissions and lower failure to discharge to home. This was especially true for trauma patients, suggesting that staffing standardization and SNF specialization may improve long-term outcomes for elderly geriatric trauma patients.

FACTORS THAT IMPAIR DISCHARGE TO HOME

Older patients have unique difficulties with recovery from surgery or injury as physiologic reserve and tolerance of adverse events decline with age. The pathophysiology of aging is believed to revolve around dysregulation of the immune, endocrine, and metabolic systems. Periods of stress, such as trauma and surgery, expose these repercussions of aging. Consequently, it is more difficult for older patients to recover, regain independence, and return home after hospital discharge.[15] Thus, helping older patients to return home requires innovative programs that go beyond reducing complication rates to enhance postoperative recovery.[16]

Preoperative or preinjury functional status is a key predictor of outcomes for older patients. Factors, such as frailty or sarcopenia, have been clearly shown to portend worse outcomes for elderly trauma and surgical patients.[17–20] Poor preoperative function is an important predictor of postoperative recovery and the need for post–acute care.[21] This is independent of the already known risk of postoperative complications among the elderly, which prolong recovery and lead to ongoing needs that require placement in post–acute care facilities. A modifiable portion of this cascade may be enhanced with prehabilitation, the process of increasing patients' functional reserve in anticipation for surgery. Although not applicable to the acutely injured or acutely ill surgical patient, prehabilitation may play an important role in elective surgical procedures in the elderly.[22] It is, therefore, important to identify high-risk patients so they can be targeted for interventions to improve recovery prior to or during the inpatient hospital stay.[23]

Although preoperative functional dependence and postoperative complications increase need for post–acute care, a retrospective study by Balentine and colleagues[16] revealed that older patients are frequently discharged to post–acute care facilities even when they are functionally independent and without postoperative complications. This study showed that patients ages 75 to 84 years who were fully independent and had an uncomplicated postoperative course were discharged to SNFs or rehabilitation hospitals 14% of the time whereas those ages 85 years and older used post–acute care facilities 30% of the time.

IMPORTANCE OF EARLY DISCHARGE PLANNING

These data strongly suggest that efforts to minimize discharge to post–acute care facilities, in particular SNFs, are important to long-term outcomes in the elderly. Potentially modifiable factors during the acute hospitalization include early mobilization, adequate nutrition, avoidance of delirium, prevention of falls, and early discharge planning.[24] In a systematic review and meta-analysis of 9 trials involving 1736 patients, Fox and colleagues[25] compared usual care to early discharge planning. These investigators found that early discharge planning was associated with fewer hospital readmissions and lower readmission lengths of hospital stay. Although there were no differences in index length of hospital stay, mortality, or satisfaction with discharge planning, several of the trials indicated that early discharge planning was associated with greater overall quality of life.

SUCCESSFUL TRANSITION OF CARE
Intradisciplinary and Interdisciplinary Communication

Frequent and clear communication among members of a patient's multidisciplinary care team serves as the groundwork for effective discharge planning and transitions of care when required. Breakdowns in communication in the acute care setting have been shown to increase patient length of stay and lead to millions of dollars in wasted resource,[26] while also having a negative impact on patient satisfaction.[27]

During a patient's hospitalization, multidisciplinary rounding can set the stage for closer communication among team members and build a group focus on successfully transitioning a patient to the next appropriate level of care. Daily rounds, however brief, have been shown to yield a significantly high rate of successfully implemented discharge plans.[28] Involvement from physicians, midlevel providers, rehabilitation services, bed coordinators, case managers and social workers, and nursing staff is key to ensuring communication flows adequately between stakeholders. A focus on the patient's current condition, recommended disposition, barriers to discharge, and next steps can align priorities and leverage the various skillsets of the multidisciplinary team. In some instances, walking rounds and the involvement of patients and families in the process may both increase patient satisfaction and reduce resource utilization after discharge.[29] Working collaboratively to avoid delays in discharge is financially advantageous and, as Rojas-García and colleagues[30] note, reduce both the physical (increased risk of decubiti and deconditioning) and emotional (anxiety and stress) tolls of discharge delays on geriatric patients.

As a patient moves toward discharge, opening a dialogue with the post–acute care providers, whether at a SNF, subacute rehabilitation, or a home health agency, can prioritize a smooth transition. Inadequate communication with facilities can ultimately lead to increased rates of hospital readmissions that seem at least partially attributable to poor care coordination. Identification of a clear plan for close follow-up care is key, and communication of this via the discharge summary can prevent an increase in readmission rates for patients discharged to subacute rehabilitation.[31] In a study by Pesko and colleagues,[32] communication breakdowns between a geriatric patient's inpatient medical team and the home health agency regarding overall plan of care and condition changes can similarly lead to an increase in readmission rates among high-risk patients. Having the hospital nursing staff give a report to each patient's accepting facility or agency on the day of discharge is another way to ensure the lines of communication are open and questions can be addressed prior to the start of care.

For patients who are discharged to their home, close collaboration with their primary care physician to clarify discharge instructions and ensure the availability of adequate follow-up care in the community may increase rates of follow-up as well as increase the likelihood a patient will complete any necessary work-ups after the acute hospitalization.[33] If geriatric patients do not have a primary care physician, connecting them to one who is easily accessible is a critical step prior to discharge.

Collaboration both horizontally and vertically through the continuum of care may be viewed as one fundamental component of a successful transition of care. Physicians and their teams who are effective in this realm provide their geriatric patients with concrete advantages in maintaining their health and staying out of the hospital.

Logistical and Practical Considerations

Even after receiving quality medical treatment, a geriatric surgical patient's successful transition of care can be derailed by a variety of systemic and psychosocial barriers. Many of these predate a patient's hospitalization, although their medical team nevertheless is required to grapple with these barriers to ensure a safe and sustainable discharge plan.

Fortunately, few geriatric patients are uninsured, with approximately 99% covered by either Medicare, Medical Assistance, private insurance, or some combination thereof.[34] Still, this does not prevent gaps in coverage from occurring. Chronically ill patients with multiple lengthy hospitalizations may run short on Medicare-covered hospital days, subacute rehabilitation or SNF days, or both. This places patients and families without a secondary insurance policy or long-term care insurance in a difficult financial position, and they are often limited in their options at the time of discharge. Furthermore, patients with limited or restricted coverage force the medical team into the difficult position of potentially forced to trade quality for cost to meet a patient's budgetary restrictions.

Geriatric patients in their initial hospitalization can be surprised by the limitations and restrictions of Medicare coverage, even when it is supplemented by a private policy. That Medicare only authorizes skilled—not custodial—services in the home, does not cover long-term care, and requires coinsurance payments beyond day 20 for subacute rehabilitation or SNF, can be a frequent source of frustration for the geriatric patient and prove a barrier for the medical team.[35] Guiding patients and their families through these limitations and helping build realistic expectations for post–acute care should become a central focus as disposition planning moves forward. Having experienced staff literate in Medicare coverage and its various limitations can ease the burden on patients who are not well versed in their options.

Early identification of financial and other social barriers is thus another key to smoothing out the geriatric patient's transition of care. Just as discharge planning begins on hospital day 1, or sometimes before, the multidisciplinary team's evaluation and intervention must begin as soon as is feasible, with a particular focus on disposition location.[9] Although Medicare does provide clear guidelines for discharge assessments,[36] going beyond these requirements to develop a holistic picture of the geriatric patient's prior level of functioning, living arrangement, family support, advance care planning, psychosocial welfare, and current and future medical needs, is key to optimizing their transition of care.[37]

Connected to this assessment process should be the early and frequent inclusion of patients and their families in decision making. Both during the hospitalization and approaching discharge, offering choice to patients, communicating regularly and predictably, and providing regular education are crucial to a focus on geriatric patient-centered care.[38] Cawthon and colleagues[39] found that bedside counseling from pharmacists trained specifically in health communication strategies was viewed as very helpful by patients, in particular those with low health literacy. A qualitative study of the elderly and disabled by Baxter and Glendinning[40] emphasized that the desire for choice, education, and timely information were common themes among these patients when being connected to social and health resources. The investigators also note the trust that this population often places in their health care and service providers when discussing these decisions. The involvement of geriatric patients or, in the case of incapacity or patient choice, their families in their own transitions of care is thankfully now common in most settings but is nevertheless worth emphasizing as a core component of disposition planning that may simultaneously increase patient satisfaction and reduce rehospitalizations.[41]

There is no singular solution to ensure a successful transition of care, particularly as patient complexity increases and staffing and resources shrink. Some suggestions for a successful transition are listed in **Box 1**. As Hansen and colleagues[42] note, a holistic approach with multiple layers of intervention both predischarge and postdischarge is likely necessary to best serve the ever-increasing population of injured and surgical geriatric patients.

Box 1
Successful transition of care

- Begins at the time of the admission and includes an early assessment of needs and barriers
- Requires multidisciplinary input
- Involves patients and families in planning
- Requires clear communication between involved members of the team
- Must include extensive patient and family education
- Thorough information transfer between hospital and discharge facility must occur
- Should be a multifaceted and holistic approach

SUMMARY

To ensure a smooth transition of care for injured and postsurgical elderly patients, early and multidisciplinary discharge planning, including not only the heath care team but also the patient and family, is increasingly recognized as paramount to this process. The same principle of open and early communication should be extended to post–acute care providers, which both decreases the burden of transfer to the patient and reduces readmissions to acute care facilities. As the population of elderly increase, it is owed to patients to not only focus on their acute medical needs during the index hospitalization but also provide them with an effective transition of care.

REFERENCES

1. US Census Bureau Statistical Brief. Economics and statistics administration, U.S. Department of Commerce. Sixty-five plus in the United States. 2011. Available at: https://www.census.gov/population/socdemo/statbriefs/agebrief.html. Accessed April 15, 2018.
2. American Hospital Association. When I'm 64: how boomers will change health care. Chicago: 2007. Available at: https://www.aha.org/system/files/content/00-10/070508-boomerreport.pdf. Accessed September 9, 2018.
3. Center for Disease Control and Prevention. Injury prevention & control: data & statistics. Available at: www.cdc.gov/injury/wisqars/pdf/leading causes of death by age group 2012-a.pdf. Accessed April 10, 2018.
4. Kozar RA, Arbabi S, Stein D, et al. Injury in the aged: geriatric trauma care at the crossroads. J Trauma Acute Care Surg 2015;78(6):1197–209.
5. Strosberg DS, Housley BC, Vazquez D, et al. Discharge destination and readmission rates in older trauma patients. J Surg Res 2017;207:27–32.
6. Claridge JA, Leukhardt WH, Golob JF, et al. Moving beyond traditional measurement of mortality after injury: evaluation of risks for late death. J Am Coll Surg 2010;210(5):788–94.
7. Richmond TS, Kauder D, Strumpf N, et al. Characteristics and outcomes of serious traumatic injury in older adults. J Am Geriatr Soc 2002;50:215–22.
8. Aitken LM, Burmeister E, Lang J, et al. Characteristics and outcomes of injured older adults after hospital admission. J Am Geriatr Soc 2010;58(3):442–9.
9. Beaulieu RA, McCarthy MC, Markert RJ, et al. Predictive factors and models for trauma patient disposition. J Surg Res 2014;190(1):264–9.
10. Ayoung-Chee P, McIntyre L, Ebel BE, et al. Long-term outcomes of ground-level falls in the elderly. J Trauma Acute Care Surg 2014;76(2):498–503.
11. Balentine CJ, Naik AD, Robinson CN, et al. Association of high-volume hospitals with greater likelihood of discharge to home following colorectal surgery. JAMA Surg 2014;149(3):244–51.
12. Sacks GD, Lawson EH, Dawes AJ, et al. Which patients require more care after hospital discharge? an analysis of post-acute care use among elderly patients undergoing elective surgery? J Am Coll Surg 2015;220(6):1113–21.
13. Hakkarainen TW, Arbabi S, Willis MM, et al. Outcomes of patients discharged to skilled nursing facilities after acute care hospitalizations. Ann Surg 2016;263(2): 280–5.
14. Thornblade LW, Arbabi S, Flum DR, et al. Facility-level factors and outcomes after skilled nursing facility admission for trauma and surgical patients. J Am Med Dir Assoc 2018;19(1):70–6.

15. Li LT, Barden GM, Balentine CJ, et al. Postoperative transitional care needs in the elderly: an outcome of recovery associated with worse long-term survival. Ann Surg 2015;261(4):695–701.

16. Balentine CJ, Naik AD, Berger DH, et al. Postacute care after major abdominal surgery in elderly patients, intersection of age, functional status and postoperative complications. JAMA Surg 2016;151(8):759–66.

17. Joseph B, Orouji Jokar T, Hassan A, et al. Redefining the association between old age and poor outcomes after trauma: the impact of frailty syndrome. J Trauma Acute Care Surg 2017;82(3):575–81.

18. Joseph B, Zangbar B, Pandit V, et al. Emergency general surgery in the elderly: too old or too frail? J Am Coll Surg 2016;222(5):805–13.

19. Afilalo J, Lauck S, Kim DH, et al. Frailty assessment in the cardiovascular care of older adults. J Am Coll Cardiol 2014;63:747–62.

20. Moisey LL, Mourtzakis M, Cotton BA, et al. Skeletal muscle predicts ventilator-free days, ICU-free days, and mortality in elderly ICU patients. Crit Care 2013;17(5): R206.

21. Lawrence VA, Hazuda HP, Cornell JE, et al. Functional independence after major abdominal surgery in the elderly. J Am Coll Surg 2004;199(5):762–72.

22. Mayo NE, Feldman L, Scott S, et al. Impact of preoperative change in physical function on postoperative recovery: argument supporting prehabilitation for colorectal surgery. Surgery 2011;150(3):505–14.

23. Cheema FN, Abraham NS, Berger DH, et al. Novel approaches to perioperative assessment and intervention may improve long-term outcomes after colorectal cancer resection in older adults. Ann Surg 2011;253(5):867–74.

24. Yeh DD, Fuentes E, Quraishi SA, et al. Adequate nutrition may get you home: effect of caloric/protein deficits on the discharge destination of critically ill surgical patients. JPEN J Parenter Enteral Nutr 2016;40(1):37–44.

25. Fox MT, Persaud M, Maimets I, et al. Effectiveness of early discharge planning in acutely ill or injured hospitalized older adults: a systematic review and meta-analysis. BMC Geriatr 2013;13:70.

26. Agarwal R, Sands D, Schneider J. Quantifying the economic impact of communication inefficiencies in U.S. hospitals. J Healthc Manag 2010;55(4):265–81.

27. Wanzer M, Booth-Butterfield M, Gruber K. Perceptions of health care providers' communication: relationships between patient-centered communication and satisfaction. Health Commun 2004;16(3):363–83.

28. Sen A, Xiao Y, Lee SA, et al. Daily multidisciplinary discharge rounds in a trauma center: a little time, well spent. J Trauma 2009;66(3):880–7.

29. Wrobleski D, Joswiak M, Dunn D, et al. Discharge planning rounds to the bedside: a patient- and family- centered approach. Medsurg Nurs 2014;23(2): 111–6.

30. Rojas-García A, Turner S, Pizzo E, et al. Impact and experiences of delayed discharge: a mixed-studies systematic review. Health Expect 2018;21(1):41–56.

31. Gilmore-Bykovskyi A, Kennelty K, DuGoff E, et al. Hospital discharge documentation of a designated clinician for follow-up care and 30-day outcomes in hip fracture and stroke patients discharged to sub-acute care. BMC Health Serv Res 2018;18(1):103.

32. Pesko M, Gerber L, Peng T, et al. Home health care: nurse-physician communication, patient severity, and hospital readmission. Health Serv Res 2018;53(2): 1008–24.

33. Balaban RB, Weissman JS, Samuel PA, et al. Redefining and redesigning hospital discharge to enhance patient care: a randomized controlled study. J Gen Intern Med 2008;23(8):1228–33.
34. United States Census Bureau. Health insurance coverage in the United States: 2015. Available at: https://www.census.gov/content/dam/Census/library/publications/2016/demo/p60-257.pdf. Accessed April 11, 2018.
35. Anderson Z. Solving America's long-term care financing crisis: financing universal long-term care insurance with mandatory federal income tax surcharge that increases with age. Elder Law J 2018;25(2):473–514.
36. Centers for Medicare and Medicaid Services. Revision to State Operations Manual (SOM), Hospital appendix A - interpretive guidelines for 42 CFR 482.43, discharge planning. Available at: https://www.cms.gov/Medicare/Provider-Enrollment-and-Certification/SurveyCertificationGenInfo/Downloads/Survey-and-Cert-Letter-13-32.pdf. Accessed April 11, 2018.
37. Holm S, Mu K. Discharge planning for the elderly in acute care: the perceptions of experienced occupational therapists. Phys Occup Ther Geriatr 2012;30(3):214–28.
38. Hanson H, Warkentin L, Wilson R, et al. Facilitators and barriers of change toward an elder-friendly surgical environment: perspectives of clinician stakeholder groups. BMC Health Serv Res 2017;17(1):1–12.
39. Cawthon C, Walia S, Osborn C, et al. Improving care transitions: the patient perspective. J Health Commun 2012;17:312–24.
40. Baxter K, Glendinning C. Making choices about support services: disabled adults' and older people's use of information. Health Soc Care Community 2011;19(3):272–9.
41. Bauer M, Fitzgerald L, Haesler E, et al. Hospital discharge planning for frail older people and their family. Are we delivering best practice? A review of the evidence. J Clin Nurs 2009;18:2539–46.
42. Hansen LO, Young RS, Hinami K, et al. Interventions to reduce 30-day rehospitalization: a systematic review. Ann Intern Med 2011;155:520–8.

Surgical Oncology and Geriatric Patients

Michael E. Johnston II, MD, Jeffrey J. Sussman, MD,
Sameer H. Patel, MD*

KEYWORDS

- Geriatric medicine • Surgical oncology • Cancer • Elderly • Treatment

KEY POINTS

- Frailty assessment should be used in the preoperative assessment of surgical oncology patients.
- Geriatric surgical oncology treatment regimens should be tailored to patients based on life expectancy, quality of life and outcomes from a surgical management.
- Research studies should incorporate and specifically stratify care in elderly patients to continue advancement of this field.

INTRODUCTION

The incidence of cancer in geriatric patients is increasing each year with currently 15.1% of the population being older than 65 years and that number is expected to increase to 21.4% in 2050.[1] Of the greater than 35 million people in the United States older than 65 years, more than 5 million are older than 80 years.[2] More than two-thirds of cancers are diagnosed in the elderly, which is expected to increase to 70% in the next 30 years. The increases in cancer incidence, life expectancy, and reduction in cardiac-related deaths have made cancer care in geriatrics an essential field.

With increasing incidence and prevalence of cancer in the elderly, emphasis has been placed on understanding their surgical management. Unfortunately, management of surgical oncology patients is complex, complicated by decreased patient physiologic reserve, multiple medical comorbidities, incorporation of novel treatment strategies, and lack of studies focusing on elderly patients.

Although the number of geriatric surgical oncology patients has been expanding, there is still a paucity of data in this patient population. This lack of data is due in part to reluctance by clinicians to incorporate elderly patients into clinical trials

Disclosure: The authors have nothing to disclose.
Department of Surgery, University of Cincinnati College of Medicine, 231 Albert Sabin Way, ML 0558, Cincinnati, OH 45267-0558, USA
* Corresponding author.
E-mail address: Patel5se@ucmail.uc.edu

Clin Geriatr Med 35 (2019) 53–63
https://doi.org/10.1016/j.cger.2018.08.006
0749-0690/19/© 2018 Elsevier Inc. All rights reserved.
geriatric.theclinics.com

because of their multiple comorbidities and suspected poor outcomes. To fill this gap, studies are now focusing on the multifactorial complexity of aging and stratifying patients based on age to identify specific issues. Furthermore, tools such as the geriatric and frailty assessment scores have been used to broaden applicability of studies with younger patients to the elderly.

Although greater lifetime exposure to carcinogens and resultant accumulation of genetic mutations is thought to be one of the major risk factors for cancer development, the biological mechanisms leading to susceptibility are not completely known. Studies have found that elderly patients have a decrease in their DNA mismatch repair system, increases in microsatellite instability with relative immunosuppression, and greater systemic susceptibility to tumor progression in comparison to younger patients.[3] Furthermore, there are differences in tumor biology, including DNA ploidy, receptor expression, and tumor progression. These apparent biological differences do not necessarily translate to affect clinical management but hint at classifying cancers based on age. Despite these differences, surgery-specific outcomes in breast, esophagogastric, colorectal, and hepatobiliary cancer are equivalent in comparison with younger patients.[4] This review discusses preoperative assessments with accompanying interventions, surgical management, advances in surgical technology, and ethical issues encountered in geriatric surgical oncology patients.

SURGICAL ONCOLOGICAL GERIATRIC ASSESSMENTS AND PREOPERATIVE OPTIMIZATION

Although frailty assessment and management in the preoperative phase has been recommended by the American College of Surgeons (ACS), many physicians use age as the sole predictor for risk, which has been proven to be unreliable.

Frailty is defined as a combination of multiple comorbidities and clinical evidence of end-organ dysfunction, which makes patients vulnerable to physiologic stressors.[5] There are multiple ways to assess frailty with more than 70 tools, ranging from a single to 70+ variable assessments. Unfortunately, because of the many available frailty assessment options, research efforts have been limited by the lack of consistency. Overall, the goal of these tools is to define frailty and predict postoperative complications.

The gold standard supported by the American Geriatric Society is the Comprehensive Geriatric Assessment (CGA).[6] The CGA is a multidisciplinary evaluation including the assessment of physical, mental, social, economic, functional, and environmental aspects of the elderly but is impractical because of the required hours to complete. An alternative, endorsed by the ACS, is the modified Frailty Index (mFI) based on the original Frailty Index by the Canadian Health and Aging Study. The mFI is a simplified index with only 11 variables (**Box 1**) and was created based on data from the National Surgical Quality Improvement Program database.[7] The mFI has been found to be predictive of intensive care–level complications, along with mortality and morbidity in surgical subspecialties. Phenotypic frailty is another utility recognized by the ACS as an optimal strategy for geriatric surgical assessment.[5] This utility uses 5 criteria, including exhaustion, gait speed, weakness, activity level, and weight loss.

While there are multiple modalities for defining frailty, there are very few studies examining ways to improve patients' frailty. Many have started to use a multimodal approach following identification of frail patients. Hall and colleagues[8] found that by simply notifying the surgeon, anesthesiologist, critical care, and palliative care teams that a patient was frail resulted in reduced patient mortality. There was no intervention aside from physician notification, which showed that increased communication

---

Box 1
The modified frailty index

History of diabetes mellitus

History of congestive heart failure

HTN requiring medication

History of TIA or CVA

Nonindependent functional status

History of myocardial infarction

History of either PVD or rest pain

History of CVA with neurologic deficit

History of COPD or pneumonia

History of PCI, PCS, or angina

History of impaired sensorium

Abbreviations: COPD, chronic obstructive pulmonary disease; CVA, cerebrovascular accident; HTN, hypertension; PCI, percutaneous coronary intervention; PCS, prior cardiac surgery; PVD, peripheral vascular disease; TIA, transischemic attack.

---

between team members can result in improved patient care and outcomes. Upon identifying frailty, the utilization of prehabilitation programs has shown to improve cardiopulmonary reserve in cardiothoracic patients, with similar improvement in physiologic reserve in surgical oncology patients; however, it has not translated to a decrease in morbidity or mortality.[9] In addition to prehabilitation and multimodal patient management, the American Geriatrics Society (AGS) recommends regional anesthesia when possible to decrease postoperative complications related to general anesthesia.[10] Furthermore, ice, local anesthesia, and reduction of narcotic use can decrease delirium, length of hospital stay, and morbidity.

BREAST CANCER

Sixty percent of breast cancer cases arise in patients older than 65 years and greater than 30% in patients older than 70 years.[11] Breast cancer surgery has been considered safe in the elderly (**Table 1**), but the overall management is controversial. Almost half of elderly patients with early breast cancer are not treated with currently available hormonal, chemotherapy, or radiotherapy, which has led to poorer prognosis and survival.[12] Studies have proven that older patients typically have more favorable cancer phenotypes for hormonotherapy (estrogen and progesterone receptor positive), decreased aggressive nature of cancer, and a lower impact on overall survival (OS).[13] These findings, in combination with multiple comorbidities in the elderly, have led physicians to favor conservative management approaches. However, with regard to surgery, the American College of Cardiology reports breast cancer operations as low risk. Furthermore, with advances in anesthesia and surgical technique, the rate of perioperative mortality has decreased. A Cochrane meta-analysis examining tamoxifen alone versus surgery (with or without tamoxifen) found worse progression-free survival but not OS in medically fit older patients who did not have surgery.[14]

Current guidelines recommend performing a sentinel lymph node (SLN) biopsy (SLNB) for patients with invasive breast cancer and clinically negative axilla. If SLNB is negative, there is no treatment necessary for the axilla. If however, the SLNB proves

Table 1
Outcome studies of breast cancer in the elderly

Author, Year	Number	Study	Outcomes	OS
Bouchardy et al,[12] 2001	Txt 1989–99	R	Poor general health, 17% of women	NR
	407 women with breast cancer		Suboptimal treatment, approximately 50%	
Donker et al,[18] 2014	744 ALND	RCT	86.9% 5-y DFS	93.3% 5 y
	681 radiotherapy		82.7% 5-y DFS	92.5% 5 y
Giuliano et al,[16] 2010	446 SNB alone	R	—	92.5% 5 y
	445 SNB + ALND			91.9% 5 y
Kunkler et al,[19] 2015	658 BCS only	RCT	4.1% 5-y recurrence	NR
	668 BCS + WBI		1.3% 5-y recurrence	

Abbreviations: ALND, axillary lymph node dissection; BCS, breast-conserving surgery; DFS, disease-free survival; ND, no difference; OS, overall survival; R, retrospective study; RCT, randomized controlled trial; SLNB, sentinel lymph node biopsy; Txt, Treated.

the presence of axillary disease, the management is still controversial; recent studies have favored conservative operative approaches in the elderly in order to reduce post-operative complications. Studies using the National Cancer Database have found that axillary lymph node dissection (ALND) is routinely omitted in patients older than 80 years.[15] Based on the ACS Oncology Group Z0011 trial,[16] patients with T1-2N0M0 breast cancer undergoing breast-conserving surgery and adjuvant whole-breast radiotherapy who were found to have 1 to 2 positive SLNs can forgo completion ALND. No difference in OS was seen in patients undergoing observation versus those undergoing ALND. When applying the Z0011 data to elderly patients, studies have similarly found no improvement in OS. Furthermore, there is suggestion that SLNB can be omitted in early stage breast cancer in the elderly because of the low incidence of axillary disease in this population.[17] In patients with positive SLNB, based on the European Organization for Research and Treatment of Cancer's AMAROS trial, axillary radiotherapy is comparable with ALND in elderly patients for axillary control with no palpable adenopathy.[18]

Multiple studies have shown that in patients undergoing breast-conserving therapy, adjuvant whole-breast radiation decreases local recurrence in patients older than 65 years.[18] However, given the low rate of ipsilateral breast cancer recurrence, there is likely a subset of patients whereby whole-breast radiotherapy can be safely omitted.[19]

GASTRIC, ESOPHAGEAL, AND ESOPHAGOGASTRIC CANCER

Most gastric cancer occurs in patients older than 65 years and many series have found that age is not a contraindication to the use of gastrectomy and lymph node dissection in elderly patients.[20] The safety and feasibility of laparoscopic gastrectomy (LG) in the elderly is proven and can reduce postoperative complications compared with open approaches.[21] A meta-analysis by Pan and colleagues[21] showed that elderly patients have no significant differences in surgical complications in comparison with younger patients undergoing LG. It did show however, that elderly patients have higher nonsurgical postoperative complications, greater delay in bowel function, and longer hospital stay. This finding is similar to the results by Zhou and colleagues,[20] which showed greater perioperative morbidity and pulmonary complications with advanced age (Table 2).[22] Kunisaki and colleagues[23] showed that elderly patients, despite having higher American of Anesthesiologist scores, were found to have similar OS when

Table 2				
Outcome studies of gastric and esophageal cancer in the elderly				
Author, Year	Study	Number	Complications (%)	OS
Gastric				
Zhou et al,[20] 2016+	R	389 <65 y	15.4% C	NR
		301 = 65–75 y	24.9% C	
		39 >75 y	48.7% C	
Takeshita et al,[22] 2013	R	1089 <80 y	29.7% C	70% 5.5 y
		104 >80 y	32.7% C	40% 5.5 y
Esophageal				
Cijs et al,[28] 2010	R	250 >70 y	17%	27% at 5 y
		811 <70 y	20%	34% at 5 y
Finlayson et al,[29] 2007	R	65–69 y	8.8% ORM	Total 27,957 pxs
		70–79 y	13.4% ORM	
		80 + y	19.9% ORM	

Abbreviations: C, complications; ND, no difference; NR, not reported; ORM, operating room mortality; Pxs, patients; R, retrospective study; RCT, randomized control trial.

compared with younger patients for LGs. When examining prognostic factors for OS, tumor size and stage but not operative approach were significant.

Adjuvant chemotherapy has shown to improve OS and disease-free survival for patients with resectable gastric cancer.[24] However, the routine use of adjuvant chemotherapy in the elderly is controversial. A meta-analysis by Chang and colleagues[25] showed there was no significant improvement in OS in the elderly receiving adjuvant chemotherapy. The authors go on to suggest that adverse events related to systemic therapy limited its use and a survival benefit may not exist for all elderly patients.

Like gastric cancer, esophageal cancer affects the geriatric population with greater than 30% of cases arising in patients older than 70 years.[26] Although early T1a lesions can be treated with less invasive endoscopic mucosal resections, elderly patients often present with more advanced disease.[27] Esophagectomy for cancer in the elderly has shown to have higher perioperative cardiovascular/respiratory complications and higher operative and in-hospital mortality.[28] Furthermore, the increased mortality after esophagectomy is directly related to age as well as surgeon expertise and volume.[29]

Neoadjuvant chemoradiotherapy using the CROSS trial (Cincinnati Research on Outcomes and Safety in Surgery) data has been the standard of care for esophageal cancer.[30] The CROSS trial had patient ages ranging from 36 to 79 years with a median age of 60 years. Although there were patients older than 65 years in the study, there is questionable applicability of the outcomes in patients older than 79 years. Despite that, studies that have examined neoadjuvant therapy specifically in elderly patients have found similar adverse event profiles and survival benefits.[31] With appropriate patient selection, risk stratification, and advances in minimally invasive esophageal surgery, esophagectomies can be performed safely with improved patient outcomes.

COLORECTAL CANCER

The Association of Coloproctology of Great Britain and Ireland study found that there was a drastic increase in mortality from colorectal cancer (CRC) seen with increasing patient age after elective colorectal surgery (likelihood of death age 65–74 years, 1.8 times; 75–84 years, 3.5 times; >85 years, 5.0 times).[32] These data suggest that surgery for CRC is not without significant risk; however, for stages I to III CRC, age is not a contraindication to surgery. Other studies in contrast have shown that despite an increased risk of perioperative morbidity, long-term survival remains equivalent between the young and old.[33] These data highlight that patient selection is an important component in the surgical decision-making process, as perioperative morbidity and mortality are major concerns.

For stage IV CRC cancer, surgery is indicated not only for bleeding, obstruction, and perforation, but also for resectable metastatic disease.[34] Studies evaluating the efficacy of CRC liver metastasis resection in the elderly have found 5-year OS ranging from 31.0% to 34.1% and mortality ranging from 4% to 7%.[35] However, the decision to operate for stage IV CRC should be based on determining the extent of the resection, patient comorbidities, and overall expected improvement in survival.

Up to 40% of elderly patients with CRC present emergently and older patients with obstructive symptoms have 3 times higher mortality in comparison with younger cohorts.[36] The use of either emergent surgery or bridging therapy with self-expanding metal stents for gastrointestinal obstruction is still debated. Outcomes after emergent surgery versus stenting and future surgery have mixed results, but a Cochrane review comparing the two found no difference in mortality or morbidity rates.[37] In these challenging cases, patient preferences, performance status, and lifestyle should be weighed against outcomes.[36]

Laparoscopic surgery for CRC has shown reductions in overall morbidity, mortality, and hospital stay compared with open surgery (**Table 3**).[38–41] Furthermore, elderly patients undergoing elective laparoscopic surgery have similar 5-year OS compared with younger patients.[21] Despite similar survival, older patients do have a higher rate of cardiac and pulmonary complications and similar rates of anastomotic leaks or reoperation.[42]

When examining systemic therapy for CRC, elderly patient are more likely to receive suboptimal treatments due to concern for poor tolerance.[43] The AGS recommends using the Chemotherapy Risk Assessment Scale for High-Age Patients (CRASH), which estimates the patients' anticipated tolerance to the chemotherapy. In addition, studies

Table 3
Outcome studies of colon and rectal cancer in the elderly

Author, Year	Number	Study	Complications (%)	OS
Colon				
Hamaker et al,[40] 2014	20,437 <75 y	L	—	0.8% Mortality at 1 y
	12,817 >75 y			2.1% Mortality at 1 y
Guo et al,[38] 2011	34 SEMS	R	—	3% Acute mortality
	58 Primary surgery			11% Acute mortality
Rectal				
Rutten et al,[41] 2008	1126 <75 y	R	8.2% Mortality after leak	—
	230 >75 y		57% Mortality after leak	
Jung et al,[39] 2009	6042 <75 y	R	8% Local recurrence	73% Cancer-specific survival
	3663 >75 y		9% Local recurrence	78% Cancer-specific survival

Abbreviations: L, laparoscopy versus open; R, retrospective study; SEMS, self-expanding metal stent.

have found that certain chemotherapies, like 5-fluoruracil, are better tolerated than oxaliplatin in the elderly.[44]

In rectal cancer, studies have shown that neoadjuvant therapy is well tolerated in the elderly and similarly provides long-term survival benefits in combination with total mesorectal excision.[45] Neoadjuvant therapy also has additional benefits, particularly in patients who have a pathologic complete response from therapy. These patients can potentially avoid surgery and the associated morbidities, particularly if the life expectancy from their general medical condition is greater than the risk of recurrence without definitive resection. However, compared with younger patients, elderly patients have increased late side effects, such as bowel-related complications, anorectal function, and fecal incontinence.[46] Surgery for CRC in the elderly is safe and can provide durable long-term survival benefits in carefully selected patients.

HEPATOBILIARY CANCER

The incidence of hepatopancreatobiliary malignancy has been rising with most cases occurring in patients in their sixth to 8 decade of life.[47] The mainstay of treatment of these patients is resection in combination with adjuvant and neoadjuvant therapies. Hepatocellular cancer (HCC) is one of the most common causes of death from cancer in the world.[48] Early studies have reported increased mortality in the elderly with hepatic resection; but recent studies, with better patient selection and improvement in surgical techniques, have shown operative mortality rates as low as 5%.[49] Although perioperative mortality rates are low, 5-year OS following hepatic resection in the elderly still varies greatly from 18% to 76%.

Kaibori and colleagues[50] showed that elderly patients with HCC have a higher incidence of underlying liver disease, predisposing them to higher perioperative complications and poorer outcomes. Laparoscopic liver resection can potentially reduce morbidity and in carefully selected patients, provide outcomes similar to younger cohorts, with no significant differences in postoperative morbidity or mortality.[51] In settings where patients are not candidates for resection, alternative treatment modalities, such as liver-directed or ablative therapy, can be used to treat the disease while removing the risks associated with surgery.

The incidence of pancreatic cancer increases proportionally with age, with average age of diagnosis being 72 years.[52] Multiple studies have shown age is not a contraindication to resection; but a Surveillance Epidemiology End Result analysis found resection for pancreatic cancer decreases proportionally with age, independent of comorbidity status.[53] For those elderly patients who do undergo surgery, morbidity rates are reported to be as high as 40% with a 5-year OS of 15% to 20%.[54] In an effort to reduce complications, studies have found that prehabilitation programs and improved patient selection can result in better outcomes, even in octogenarians.

MINIMALLY INVASIVE SURGERY IN GERIATRIC SURGICAL ONCOLOGY

Minimally invasive surgery (MIS) using either laparoscopic or robotic techniques has been shown to reduce wound size and potential damage to the body resulting in decreased physiologic stress in comparison with open surgery.[55] Studies have found an association with the reduction in stress of MIS with decreased complication rates, length of stay, intensive-care-unit admission, and mortality.[56] In elderly patients, it is thought that by reducing physiologic stress from surgery, frail patients are not pushed over the frailty threshold and are more likely to recover with less complications.[5]

Unfortunately, there are limited data specifically focusing on MIS in geriatric surgical oncology patients.

ETHICS IN MANAGEMENT OF GERIATRIC SURGICAL ONCOLOGY PATIENTS

In solid tumors, surgery provides the only chance for complete cure; the ultimate decision for resection lies with the surgeon. The management of geriatric patients adds an additional layer of complexity, which must take into account the cancer type, age, frailty, surgeon preference, surgeon experience, patient values, and quality of life (QoL). Furthermore, cure needs to be discussed, as a disease-free interval beyond 5 years may be sufficient for an elderly patient but not a younger one. The competing mortality from cancer needs to be weighed against death from all other causes. Handling these multiple issues in patient care can be difficult and requires a comprehensive multidisciplinary conversation. Thorough understanding and application of the principles of ethics are required: beneficence, nonmalfeasance, autonomy, and justice.[57]

The Surgical Task Force at the International Society for Geriatric Oncology performed a survey to assess the surgical oncologist's management of geriatric patients. They reported that QoL was the most important factor in the determination of a surgeon's preference on whether to operate, whereas elderly patients placed greater emphasis on the ability to maintain continued independence and health.[58] There is evidence that QoL is a definition that varies across age ranges and per patient. A physician needs to have the ability to discuss with patients their personal goals in addition to the clinical goals of care.

Palliative care is increasingly used in medical practice, but surgery as a field has been slower in incorporating its use.[59] Palliative care not only pertains to end-of-life care but encompasses treatments that focus on improving QoL rather than cure through chemotherapy, radiation therapy, and surgery. The overall care of geriatric surgical oncology patients should involve a multidisciplinary approach that considers the patients' wishes as well as the clinical teams' goals in order to provide the highest level of care.

Finally, consideration must be given to understanding patients' life expectancy based on their medical comorbidities, the risk of death from not treating the cancer, and expected survival advantage with surgery. If life expectancy based on medical comorbidity is short, there may not be a benefit of aggressive surgery, particularly if the malignancy has a more indolent course. To help determine this risk, future studies should use disease-specific survival instead of OS as an end point to better stratify these groups.

SUMMARY

Geriatric surgical oncology is an expanding field with a growing impact on medicine. Despite the rapid growth, data for specific assessments, treatments, and outcomes are lacking because of the paucity of evidence-based studies focusing specifically on this patient population. Attention needs to be turned toward developing better geriatric assessment tools, preoperative optimization, incorporation of surgical technology, and greater utilization of specific geriatric multidisciplinary teams to provide higher levels of patient care.

REFERENCES

1. Soto-Perez-de-Celis E, de Glas NA, Hsu T, et al. Global geriatric oncology: achievements and challenges. J Geriatr Oncol 2017;8(5):374–86.
2. Ferrucci L, Giallauria F, Guralnik JM, et al. Epidemiology of aging. Radiol Clin North Am 2008;46(4):643–52.
3. Berger NA, Savvides P, Koroukian SM, et al. Cancer in the elderly. Trans Am Clin Climatol Assoc 2006;117:147–56.

4. Lu Q, Lu JW, Wu Z, et al. Perioperative outcome of elderly versus younger patients undergoing major hepatic or pancreatic surgery. Clin Interv Aging 2018; 13:133–41.
5. Ethun CG, Bilen MA, Jani AB, et al. Frailty and cancer: implications for oncology surgery, medical oncology, and radiation oncology. CA Cancer J Clin 2017;67(5): 362–77.
6. Extermann M, Aapro M, Bernabei R, et al. Use of comprehensive geriatric assessment in older cancer patients. Crit Rev Oncol Hematol 2005;55(3):241–52.
7. Obeid NM, Azuh O, Reddy S, et al. Predictors of critical care-related complications in colectomy patients using the national surgical quality improvement program: exploring frailty and aggressive laparoscopic approaches. J Trauma Acute Care Surg 2012;72(4):878–83.
8. Hall DE, Arya S, Schmid KK, et al. Association of a frailty screening initiative with postoperative survival at 30, 180, and 365 days. JAMA Surg 2017;152(3):233–40.
9. Hijazi Y, Gondal U, Aziz O. A systematic review of prehabilitation programs in abdominal cancer surgery. Int J Surg 2017;39:156–62.
10. Mohanty S, Rosenthal RA, Russell MM, et al. Optimal perioperative management of the geriatric patient: a best practices guideline from the American College of Surgeons Nsqip and the American Geriatrics Society. J Am Coll Surg 2016; 222(5):930–47.
11. Jemal A, Ward E, Thun MJ. Recent trends in breast cancer incidence rates by age and optimal perioperative management of the geriatric patient: a best practices guideline from the American college of surgeons nsqip and the American geriatrics society tumor characteristics among U.S. women. Breast Cancer Res 2007;9(3):R28.
12. Bouchardy C, Rapiti E, Fioretta G, et al. Undertreatment strongly decreases prognosis of breast cancer in elderly women. J Clin Oncol 2003;21(19):3580–7.
13. Pappo I, Karni T, Sandbank J, et al. Breast cancer in the elderly: histological, hormonal and surgical characteristics. Breast 2007;16(1):60–7.
14. Hind D, Wyld L, Reed MW. Surgery, with or without tamoxifen, vs tamoxifen alone for older women with operable breast cancer: Cochrane review. Br J Cancer 2007;96(7):1025–9.
15. Bland KI, Scott-Conner CE, Menck H, et al. Axillary dissection in breast-conserving surgery for stage i and ii breast cancer: a national cancer data base study of patterns of omission and implications for survival11no competing interests declared. J Am Coll Surg 1999;188(6):586–95.
16. Giuliano AE, McCall LM, Beitsch PD, et al. Acosog Z0011: a randomized trial of axillary node dissection in women with clinical t1-2 n0 m0 breast cancer who have a positive sentinel node. J Clin Oncol 2010;28(18_suppl):CRA506.
17. Martelli G, Boracchi P, Ardoino I, et al. Axillary dissection versus no axillary dissection in older patients with t1n0 breast cancer: 15-year results of a randomized controlled trial. Ann Surg 2012;256(6):920–4.
18. Donker M, van Tienhoven G, Straver ME, et al. Radiotherapy or surgery of the axilla after a positive sentinel node in breast cancer (Eortc 10981-22023 Amaros): a randomised, multicentre, open-label, phase 3 non-inferiority trial. Lancet Oncol 2014;15(12):1303–10.
19. Kunkler IH, Williams LJ, Jack WJ, et al. Breast-conserving surgery with or without irradiation in women aged 65 years or older with early breast cancer (prime ii): a randomised controlled trial. Lancet Oncol 2015;16(3):266–73.
20. Zhou CJ, Chen FF, Zhuang CL, et al. Feasibility of radical gastrectomy for elderly patients with gastric cancer. Eur J Surg Oncol 2016;42(2):303–11.

21. Pan Y, Chen K, Yu WH, et al. Laparoscopic gastrectomy for elderly patients with gastric cancer: a systematic review with meta-analysis. Medicine 2018;97(8): e0007.
22. Takeshita H, Ichikawa D, Komatsu S, et al. Surgical outcomes of gastrectomy for elderly patients with gastric cancer. World J Surg 2013;37(12):2891–8.
23. Kunisaki C, Makino H, Takagawa R, et al. Efficacy of laparoscopy-assisted distal gastrectomy for gastric cancer in the elderly. Surg Endosc 2009;23(2):377–83.
24. Cunningham D, Allum WH, Stenning SP, et al. Perioperative chemotherapy versus surgery alone for resectable gastroesophageal cancer. N Engl J Med 2006; 355(1):11–20.
25. Chang S-H, Kim SN, Choi HJ, et al. Adjuvant chemotherapy for advanced gastric cancer in elderly and non-elderly patients: meta-analysis of randomized controlled trials. Cancer Res Treat 2017;49(1):263–73.
26. Seer Cancer Statistics Review, 1975-2009 (Vintage 2009 Populations). 2012.
27. Zehetner J, Lipham JC, Ayazi S, et al. Esophagectomy for cancer in octogenarians. Dis Esophagus 2010;23(8):666–9.
28. Cijs TM, Verhoef C, Steyerberg EW, et al. Outcome of esophagectomy for cancer in elderly patients. Ann Thorac Surg 2010;90(3):900–7.
29. Finlayson E, Fan Z, Birkmeyer JD. Outcomes in octogenarians undergoing high-risk cancer operation: a national study. J Am Coll Surg 2007;205(6):729–34.
30. Van Hagen P, Hulshof MC, van Lanschot JJ, et al. Preoperative chemoradiotherapy for esophageal or junctional cancer. N Engl J Med 2012;366(22):2074–84.
31. Takeuchi S, Ohtsu A, Doi T, et al. A retrospective study of definitive chemoradiotherapy for elderly patients with esophageal cancer. Am J Clin Oncol 2007;30(6): 607–11.
32. Tekkis PP, et al. ACPGBI Colorectal Cancer Study 2002: part A - unadjusted outcomes Part B - risk adjusted outcomes The ACPGBI Colorectal Cancer Model. 0000.
33. Kunitake H, Zingmond DS, Ryoo J, et al. Caring for octogenarian and nonagenarian patients with colorectal cancer: what should our standards and expectations be? Dis Colon Rectum 2010;53(5):735–43.
34. National Compreshensive Cancer Network. Available at: https://wwwnccnorg/professionals/hysician_gls/pdf/colonpdf. Accessed June 6, 2018.
35. Tanaka K, Shimada H, Matsuo K, et al. Outcome after simultaneous colorectal and hepatic resection for colorectal cancer with synchronous metastases. Surgery 2004;136(3):650–9.
36. Pavlidis TE, Marakis G, Ballas K, et al. Safety of bowel resection for colorectal surgical emergency in the elderly. Colorectal Dis 2006;8(8):657–62.
37. Sagar J. Colorectal stents for the management of malignant colonic obstructions. Cochrane Database Syst Rev 2011;(11):CD007378.
38. Guo MG, Feng Y, Zheng Q, et al. Comparison of self-expanding metal stents and urgent surgery for left-sided malignant colonic obstruction in elderly patients. Dig Dis Sci 2011;56(9):2706–10.
39. Jung B, Påhlman L, Johansson R, et al. Rectal cancer treatment and outcome in the elderly: an audit based on the Swedish rectal cancer registry 1995-2004. BMC Cancer 2009;9:68.
40. Hamaker ME, Schiphorst AH, Verweij NM, et al. Improved survival for older patients undergoing surgery for colorectal cancer between 2008 and 2011. Int J Colorectal Dis 2014;29(10):1231–6.
41. Rutten HJT, den Dulk M, Lemmens VE, et al. Controversies of total mesorectal excision for rectal cancer in elderly patients. Lancet Oncol 2008;9(5):494–501.

42. Stocchi L, Nelson H, Young-Fadok TM, et al. Safety and advantages of laparoscopic vs. open colectomy in the elderly: matched-control study. Dis Colon Rectum 2000;43(3):326–32.
43. Aparicio T, Navazesh A, Boutron I, et al. Half of elderly patients routinely treated for colorectal cancer receive a sub-standard treatment. Crit Rev Oncol Hematol 2009;71(3):249–57.
44. McCleary NJ, Meyerhardt JA, Green E, et al. Impact of age on the efficacy of newer adjuvant therapies in patients with stage ii/iii colon cancer: findings from the accent database. J Clin Oncol 2013;31(20):2600–6.
45. Manceau G, Karoui M, Werner A, et al. Comparative outcomes of rectal cancer surgery between elderly and non-elderly patients: a systematic review. Lancet Oncol 2012;13(12):e525–36.
46. Bruheim K, Guren MG, Skovlund E, et al. Late side effects and quality of life after radiotherapy for rectal cancer. Int J Radiat Oncol Biol Phys 2010;76(4):1005–11.
47. Seer Cancer Statistics Review 1975-2001. Available at: https://seercancergov/. Accessed June 6, 2018.
48. Siegel RL, Miller KD, Jemal A. Cancer statistics, 2017. CA Cancer J Clin 2017; 67(1):7–30.
49. Poon RTP, Fan ST, Lo CM, et al. Hepatocellular carcinoma in the elderly: results of surgical and nonsurgical management. Am J Gastroenterol 1999;94:2460–6.
50. Kaibori M, Ishizaki M, Matsui K, et al. Geriatric assessment as a predictor of postoperative complications in elderly patients with hepatocellular carcinoma. Langenbecks Arch Surg 2016;401(2):205–14.
51. Cauchy F, Fuks D, Nomi T, et al. Benefits of laparoscopy in elderly patients requiring major liver resection. J Am Coll Surg 2016;222(2):174–84.e10.
52. Frakes J, Mellon EA, Springett GM, et al. Outcomes of adjuvant radiotherapy and lymph node resection in elderly patients with pancreatic cancer treated with surgery and chemotherapy. J Gastrointest Oncol 2017;8(5):758–65.
53. Makary MA, Winter JM, Cameron JL, et al. Pancreaticoduodenectomy in the very elderly. J Gastrointest Surg 2006;10(3):347–56.
54. Riall TS, Cameron JL, Lillemoe KD, et al. Resected periampullary adenocarcinoma: 5-year survivors and their 6- to 10-year follow-up. Surgery 2006;140(5): 764–72.
55. Ballesta Lopez C, Cid JA, Poves I, et al. Laparoscopic surgery in the elderly patient. Surg Endosc 2003;17(2):333–7.
56. Korc-Grodzicki B, Downey RJ, Shahrokni A, et al. Surgical considerations in older adults with cancer. J Clin Oncol 2014;32(24):2647–53.
57. Daher M. Ethical issues in the geriatric patient with advanced cancer 'living to the end'. Ann Oncol 2013;24(Suppl 7):55–8.
58. Geriatric oncology: personalised medicine when you are old. Cancer World 2016; 75. Available at: http://cancerworld.net/cover-story/geriatric-oncology-personalised-medicine-when-you-are-old/.
59. Easson AM, Crosby JA, Librach SL. Discussion of death and dying in surgical textbooks. Am J Surg 2001;182(1):34–9.

Orthopedic Surgery and the Geriatric Patient

Alexander S. Greenstein, MD, John T. Gorczyca, MD*

KEYWORDS

- Orthopaedic surgery • Orthopedic surgery • Geriatric patient • Osteoporosis • Falls
- Fragility fracture • Comanagement

KEY POINTS

- The article reviews the evaluation of the geriatric patient from an orthopedic perspective.
- The article focuses on the workup and preoperative diagnostic evaluation and assessment as well as perioperative care provided to optimize outcomes.
- The article concludes with a review of the care of the geriatric orthopedic patient in the posthospital time period.
- The article reviews the diagnosis, workup, and treatment of osteoporosis.
- The article reviews medical comanagement and preoperative patient clearance before orthopedic procedures.

INTRODUCTION

There are an increasing number of geriatric patients. In 1950, approximately 8% of the world's population was 60 years and older. By 2000, this number had increased to 10%; it is expected to exceed 20% by 2030.[1,2] As more patients live longer, it is probable that an increasing number of geriatric patients will require surgery. Medical comorbidities and perioperative risk of geriatric patients become increasingly complex with time as patients live longer, even unhealthy patients. A judicious assessment of surgical indications, risks, and benefits is essential in this population. An organized, systematic, coordinated, multidisciplinary approach to the perioperative management of these patients will result in fewer complications, improved outcomes, and reduced cost of care.

This article reviews the evaluation of the geriatric patient from an orthopedic perspective. Details are provided on the preoperative diagnostic evaluation and

Disclosure Statement: The authors have nothing to disclose.
Department of Orthopaedics, University of Rochester Medical Center, 601 Elmwood Avenue, Box 665, Rochester, NY 14642, USA
* Corresponding author.
E-mail address: John_Gorczyca@URMC.Rochester.edu

assessment as well as perioperative care provided to optimize outcomes. The article concludes with a review of the care of the geriatric orthopedic patient in the posthospital time period.

PATIENT EVALUATION: EVALUATION OF THE GERIATRIC PATIENT FROM AN ORTHOPEDIC PERSPECTIVE
Osteoporosis

Osteoporosis is defined by structural loss of bone tissue and disruption of bone architecture that leads to low bone mass and is characterized by compromised bone strength, and an increased susceptibility to fractures. In the past, osteoporosis was defined as a disorder of low bone mineral density (BMD) alone, but this definition does not reflect the true significance of osteoporosis. Although osteoporosis is a disease involving bone, its presence often indicates a decline in overall health. Osteoporosis affects both sexes and all races; its prevalence will increase as the population ages. Based on data from the National Health and Nutrition Examination Survey III (NHANES III), the National Osteoporosis Foundation has estimated that more than 9.9 million Americans have osteoporosis and an additional 43.1 million have low bone density.[3] One of every 2 white women will experience an osteoporosis-related fracture at some point in her lifetime, as will one in 5 white men.[4] Although osteoporosis is less frequent in African Americans, when it is present, they have the same elevated fracture risk as whites. The total impact of osteoporosis on the orthopedic patient is enormous, and its prevalence has the ability to compromise patient outcomes on multiple fronts.

Screening for osteoporosis should generally begin in women aged 65 years and older and men 70 years and older with use of a dual-energy x-ray absorptiometry (DEXA) scan. The age for initial DEXA scan screening is reduced by 5 years for each risk factor: family history of osteoporosis or fragility fracture in a first-degree relative; active smoking; early hysterectomy; low body weight; history of fragility fracture; and use of oral corticosteroid therapy. Several studies on the treatment of osteoporosis following hip fractures have demonstrated that an unacceptably low number of these osteoporotic patients end up getting treated for osteoporosis, ranging from 5% to 30%.[5–10] It is the responsibility of the treating surgeon to assure the patient is properly screened and treated for osteoporosis. When the orthopedic surgeon initiates diagnosis and risk stratification, studies have shown the likelihood the patient will receive proper treatment increases dramatically,[11,12] emphasizing the importance of the surgeon as a physician who should treat the patient's overall health. Therefore, early diagnosis, treatment, and prevention of fragility fractures are paramount.

DEXA scans measure BMD, expressed in absolute terms as grams of mineral per square centimeter scanned (g/cm^2). BMD is considered to be the standard measure for the diagnosis of osteoporosis and the assessment of fracture risk. A patient's BMD can also be related to a reference value for young (30-year-old), healthy, nonosteoporotic adults of the same sex by using the T score. The T score is reported as the number of standard deviations that a patient's BMD value is above (+) or below (−) the average value for a healthy, nonosteoporotic 30-year-old adult. The World Health Organization (WHO) uses a T score less than −2.5 as a threshold to diagnose osteoporosis. Fracture risk increases doubles for every standard deviation below the mean for a 30-year-old adult.[13,14] It should be noted, however, that most fragility fractures occur in patients with BMD in the *osteopenic* range,[15–17] that is, a T score of −1 to −2.5. Therefore, detection of low BMD is important in predicting future fracture risk and in initiating proper treatment.

In addition to BMD, there are several other risk factors that will add to the accuracy of fracture prediction.[18] The WHO developed the Fracture Risk Assessment Tool (FRAX) to evaluate fracture risk of patients. FRAX was developed using a series of meta-analyses to combine clinical risk factors with BMD in order to improve predictive value for fracture risk.[19–21] FRAX calculates the 10-year probability of a major osteoporotic fracture (in the proximal part of the humerus, the wrist, or the hip or a clinical vertebral fracture) and of a hip fracture calibrated to the fracture and death hazards.[22,23] Of note, the calculated FRAX score risk of fracture is applicable only for patients who are not receiving osteoporosis medications. Thus, the physician should incorporate patient history, T score, and FRAX predictions in the evaluation and treatment of patients with osteoporosis.

Fragility fractures

A fragility fracture results from a fall from standing height or less. In 2005, there were nearly 2 million fragility fractures in the United States, with an expected increase to more than 3 million by 2025.[24] In 2004, the US Surgeon General released a report on bone health and osteoporosis that urged health care providers to address osteoporosis and fracture prevention. The report recognized that only one in 5 adults with fragility fractures receives treatment after fracture.[4] Despite this call to action and the significant resources put forth to increase secondary fracture prevention, the chance that a patient with osteoporosis would actually receive treatment actually worsened during the early 2000s.[25] Thus, this problem is expanding even quicker than expected, necessitating even more thorough measures in diagnosis, treatment, and prevention if we are to have an acceptable impact.

Secondary prevention programs for osteoporosis are interventions occurring after a disease-related complication, that is, fractures. There is a high rate of success in improving osteoporosis treatment after fractures, and in decreasing the rate of fracture occurrence in certain managed-care and single-payer systems.[26–29] However, in nonmanaged care environments, implementation of such programs has been less successful.[30] It is important to note that many patients (as high as 45%) who ultimately sustain a hip fracture have sustained prior fragility fractures. It has been estimated that there could be 22% fewer hip fractures if all patients with a prior fracture had been treated for osteoporosis, with an estimated savings of $3.4 million.[31] Thus, all patients with fragility fractures should be aggressively evaluated and treated for osteoporosis. In these times of increasing fiscal constraint on health care expenditures, addressing prevention is clearly beneficial and highly cost-effective by preventing future fractures.[22] Preventing fracture-related disability also improves quality of life for older adults, serving to maintain patients' physical independence, comfort, and dignity with aging.

Osteoporosis and Orthopedic Surgery

Mild to moderate osteoporosis may not be detectable on plain radiograph. The orthopedic surgeon should consider ordering a DEXA scan in geriatric patients before major elective orthopedic surgeries, such as a spine fusion or joint replacement.[32] Patients with osteoporosis are more likely to sustain fractures and to have a pathologic reaction of the osteoporotic bone to the implant. Osteopenic and osteoporotic bone necessitate consideration of technical details in order to avoid complications that are more common in osteopenic fractures, which are becoming increasingly severe and multifragmentary despite the low-energy mechanism[33,34]

(**Fig. 1**). The surgeon must be prepared to address the difficulty of maintaining reduction of fracture, whether treated nonoperatively or operatively[23,35–38]; compromised bone healing[39]; slower osteointegration of implants[38,40]; higher rates of complications; and worse patient-reported outcomes.[41]

The decreased quantity of mineralized tissue per unit volume in a patient with osteoporosis results in weaker strength of initial screw fixation; the impaired intrinsic mechanical properties of the bone lead to lower resistance to screw pullout. In addition,

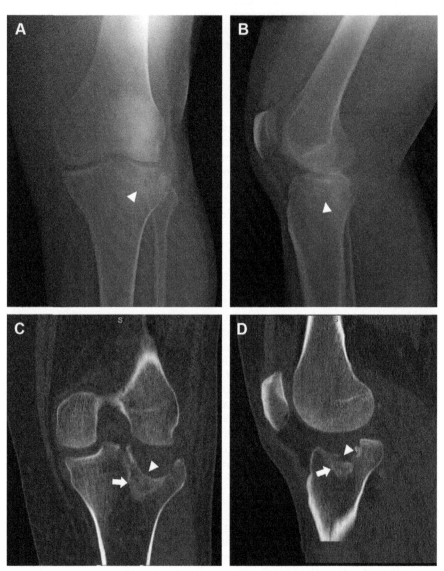

Fig. 1. Anteroposterior (AP) and lateral radiographs. AP (*A*) and lateral (*B*) radiographs of a left knee demonstrating a Schatzker 3 tibial plateau fracture with significant depression of the joint surface (*arrowheads*) from a low-energy fall. Coronal (*C*) and sagittal (*D*) CT scan cuts further demonstrating depression of the joint surface (*arrowheads*) with subchondral and metaphyseal impaction (*arrows*).

osteoporotic bone is more brittle and less elastic, rendering it even more vulnerable to iatrogenic fracture during fixation or manipulation. To address the weaker, more brittle bone, the surgeon needs to create a balance between construct stiffness and efficient load transfer to avoid stress shielding and fixation failure.[42] Osteoporotic bone may benefit from the use of materials to enhance the surrounding bony environment to enhance stability and minimize fixation failure. These materials include bone graft (cancellous or structural), bone cements, synthetic bone graft substitute, or hydroxyapatite coatings.[43,44]

Finally, osteoporotic bone may impair the patient's postoperative activity level. Although early mobilization is oftentimes the goal of surgery, most elderly patients are unable to mobilize independently without bearing full weight through the injured extremity, which may create high stresses that compromise fixation (**Fig. 2**). Orthopedists are working to develop alternative methods for geriatric and osteoporotic fragility fracture fixation to expedite weight bearing without compromising fixation.

Laboratory Assessment of Osteoporosis and Bone Health

Measurement of serum calcium, vitamin D, parathyroid hormone (PTH), testosterone, and thyroid-stimulating hormone (TSH) levels may be helpful to rule out

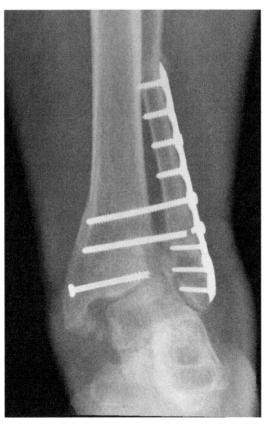

Fig. 2. AP radiograph of a left ankle demonstrating implant failure and proximal fracture of the fibula in an osteoporotic patient who bore weight before the fracture had healed.

secondary causes of osteoporosis (**Box 1**).[29,45] These laboratory tests should be ordered on all patients who have sustained a fragility fracture. Orthopedic trauma patients 50 years and older, patients with known risk factors, and patients with nonunions should also be screened. In addition, heavy consideration should be placed to ordering the aforementioned laboratory tests in the routine preoperative evaluation of geriatric patients scheduled to undergo elective arthroplasty and spine surgeries. Specialist referral is indicated for management of metabolic bone disease or testosterone replacement. The subsequent sections provide a brief overview of the laboratory studies, and their importance in management of osteoporosis and metabolic bone disease.

Vitamin D

The primary function of vitamin D is to maintain serum calcium homeostasis. The term vitamin D typically refers to *cholecalciferol* (*vitamin D3*). Calcifediol (25-hydroxyvitamin D_3) and calcitriol (1,25-dihydroxyvitamin D_3) are hydroxylated forms of vitamin D_3. Ergocalciferol (vitamin D_2), derived from plants, is a less potent form of vitamin D, which is frequently found in commercially available oral vitamins. It is also important to note vitamin D levels are reported as in either nanogram per milliliter (ng/mL) or nanomole per milliliter (nmol/L), where 1 ng/mL = 2.5 nmol/L.[46]

Recently, there has been a considerable increase in attention on vitamin D because of studies demonstrating high prevalence of vitamin D deficiency in otherwise healthy populations[47,48] as well as vitamin D's association with a multitude of clinical conditions. Vitamin D is obtained through a combination of dietary sources, oral supplements, and exposure to sunlight. In vivo conversion of 7-dehydrocholesterol to vitamin D_3 by UV-B radiation in the skin is the primary source of vitamin D in most people. Otherwise, inactive vitamin D must be hydroxylated in the liver and kidney to the active vitamin D_3. Once activated, vitamin D acts through a single, common vitamin D receptor that binds to specific DNA sequences known as vitamin D response elements, currently found on more than 200 genes in a wide distribution of tissues.[46,49] The production of 1,25-dihydroxyvitamin D is tightly regulated by a homeostatic interaction between PTH, calcium, and phosphate in the kidneys. Disease states resulting in hepatic or renal dysfunction can disrupt the vitamin D metabolic pathway and may require treatment with vitamin D_3 or 1,25-dihydroxyvitamin D_3, respectively. Thus, a complete patient assessment is necessary in the evaluation of vitamin D levels.

Universal screening of vitamin D levels and routine supplementation was found to be cost-effective in patients 65 and older.[50] The Centers for Medicare and Medicaid

---

Box 1
Laboratory evaluation of metabolic bone health

PTH

TSH

Calcium

Vitamin D

Testosterone[a]

[a] For men. Testosterone levels should be drawn between 7 AM and 10 AM.

Services have recognized counseling on vitamin D and calcium intake for the prevention of osteoporosis in patients aged 50 and older by making it a quality measure.[51] Screening for hypovitaminosis D is especially important in patients scheduled to undergo elective orthopedic surgery. Hypovitaminosis D has been identified in approximately 65% of individuals undergoing total joint arthroplasty.[52] Most recently, hypovitaminosis D was present in 97% of orthopedic trauma patients who were not already taking supplements.[53] Serum levels respond to treatment within a few weeks, but it is unclear whether the long-term effects of vitamin D deficiency can be corrected by oral supplementation alone. Vitamin D supplementation has been shown to increase the likelihood of bone healing and may reduce surgical site infection risk,[54] a devastating complication of elective orthopedic procedures. Orthopedic hardware relies on the integrity of the bone-implant interface. All of these points justify optimization of vitamin D as a means of improving patient outcomes.

The minimum target serum concentration for 25-hydroxyvitamin D should be greater than 30 ng/mL.[55] Oral supplementation of cholecalciferol (D_3) doses ranging from 400 to 2000 IU per day has been effective in treating vitamin D deficiency based on observational and randomized studies. In patients with severe deficiencies (<20 ng/mL), oral doses as high as 50,000 IU/wk are prescribed. An alternative treatment algorithm for severe deficiencies (<20 ng/mL) has been to prescribe 50,000 IU/wk of ergocalciferol (D_2) for 12 weeks and then recheck a vitamin D serum level. Daily supplementation in lower doses is thought to be superior to larger, less frequent doses, and vitamin D_3 has been shown to be more effective than vitamin D_2 in maintaining levels over time.[56–59] Overall, vitamin D is extremely safe and inexpensive, but ordinary multivitamin tablets do not provide sufficient quantities of vitamin D. Thus, universal vitamin D supplementation is crucial.

Calcium

Whether coming from diet or bones, calcium is a necessary ion for a multitude of cellular functions. Calcium constitutes approximately 2% of adult body weight, all but 1% contained in the bones, where it exists as calcium hydroxyapatite. Specifically, calcium strengthens bones through the apposition of calcium hydroxyapatite crystals to the type 1 collagen matrix that constitutes bone. The concentration of serum calcium is tightly regulated by PTH and vitamin D, with the calcium hydroxyapatite of bone serving as the largest calcium repository. Hypocalcemia, regardless of its cause, leads to a secondary hyperparathyroidism, increased bone turnover, bone loss, and increased fracture risk.[60] Therefore, adequate calcium status is imperative for bone.

Dietary calcium intake may be adequate in some individuals. Large level population estimates based on NHANES data show inadequate calcium intake from diet alone in 75% of cases, and even among supplement users, less than half of subjects achieved recommended calcium intake.[61] Calcium supplementation has been shown through meta-analysis to reduce the rate of BMD loss in both men and women[62,63] as well as to prevent fragility fractures.[64,65] The Women's Health Initiative study, which included more than 36,000 postmenopausal women, showed higher BMD at the hip in the calcium plus vitamin D group than in the placebo group.[66] In a more recent study on about 7000 subjects older than 50 years of age, a calcium intake less than 400 mg per day was associated with lower BMD and femoral cortical thickness, whereas a calcium intake greater than 1200 mg per day was positively correlated with BMD.[67]

Taken together, the literature suggests calcium supplementation has positive effects on BMD and reduces the risk of fractures. If a patient is found to be osteoporotic or sustains a fragility fracture and does not have any contraindications, calcium supplementation should be started alongside vitamin D. Recommended calcium supplement doses range from 500 to 1200 mg daily.[66,68–74] Moreover, there is a paucity of literature examining supplementation in premenopausal women and in men with osteoporosis. In line with the literature, postmenopausal women are recommended to take 1200 mg daily of elemental calcium in divided doses; men and premenopausal women with osteoporosis are recommended to supplement with 1000 mg daily in divided doses.

Parathyroid hormone
PTH, which is produced and secreted by the parathyroid glands, is an important regulator of calcium homeostasis. PTH promotes reabsorption of calcium in the renal nephron, activation of 1-hydroxylase in the kidney to produce the active metabolite of vitamin D (1,25-dihydroxyvitamin D), and resorption of calcium from bone. Although intermittent, pulsatile PTH is associated with bone deposition, chronically elevated PTH is a common cause of decreased BMD. If elevated PTH levels are identified on screening, the cause should be identified and treated as otherwise the hyperparathyroidism will lead to significantly increased bone turnover.

Testosterone
Testosterone takes part in building the skeleton of young men and in helping to prevent bone loss in elderly men. Normal testosterone levels vary, and testosterone levels decrease with aging. Even among otherwise healthy men, BMD declines from age 20 to age 90 in the femur and spine.[75] The orthopedic surgeon should refer the patient to a metabolic bone specialist for treatment if a patient with low testosterone is identified.

Thyroid stimulating hormone
TSH levels are a utilitarian method of screening for thyroid dysfunction and may identify easily treated causes of metabolic bone derangements. Thyroid hormone has a wide range of effects throughout the human body, including direct and indirect actions on osteoblasts and osteoclasts.[76–78] It stimulates bone resorption through direct action on osteoclasts, and by acting on osteoblasts, which in turn indirectly mediate osteoclastic bone resorption.[79,80] These effects, which dysregulate mineral metabolism, cause secondary and tertiary concerns in the osteoporotic patient. The hypercalcemia in patients with hyperthyroidism suppresses secretion of PTH, which allows for hypercalciuria. Although this hypercalciuria is an attempt at protecting against hypercalcemia, a net negative calcium balance results. Hypercalcemia also suppresses the secretion of PTH, reducing the conversion to the active form of vitamin D (1,25-dihydroxyvitamin D). Vitamin D metabolism is also directly increased by hyperthyroidism.[81] Thus, the direct and indirect effects of hyperthyroidism result in calcium wasting and further demineralization of bone. For these reasons, evaluation and treatment of thyroid disorders are imperative in the orthopedic patient.

Pharmacologic Treatment of Osteoporosis
Pharmacologic treatment of osteoporosis is indicated in the following patients[82,83]:

1. Those with T scores ≤ -2.5 at the femoral neck, total hip or lumbar spine by DEXA, which defines osteoporosis
2. Those with hip or vertebral (clinical or asymptomatic) fractures
3. In postmenopausal women and men aged 50 and older with low bone mass (T score between −1.0 and −2.5, osteopenia) at the femoral neck, total hip, or lumbar spine by DXA and 10-year hip fracture probability $\geq 3\%$ or a 10-year major osteoporosis-related fracture probability $\geq 20\%$ based on the US-adapted WHO absolute fracture risk model.

Pharmacologic agents include calcium and vitamin D, bisphosphonates, calcitonin, raloxifene, teriparatide, and denosumab. Conjugated estrogen-progestin hormone replacement, estrogen-only replacement have been used in the past, but have fallen out of favor due to recognition of their risks of thromboembolism and general tolerability and efficacy of other agents. The following sections briefly touch on bisphosphonates, teriparatide, and denosumab.

Bisphosphonates

Bisphosphonates are a class of drugs that inhibit osteoclast resorption, thereby preventing bone loss. There are 2 classes of bisphosphonates: nitrogen containing and nonnitrogen containing. Nitrogen-containing bisphosphonates inhibit osteoclast farnesyl pyrophosphate synthase in the mevalonate (cholesterol) pathway. Inhibition of the mevalonate pathway leads to cytoskeletal abnormalities in the osteoclast causing it to detach from the bone perimeter, ultimately resulting in less bone resorption.[84–87] Non-nitrogen-containing bisphosphonates are metabolized by osteoclasts causing osteoclasts to undergo premature death and apoptosis by forming a toxic adenosine triphosphate analogue.[86]

Regardless of choice between nitrogen-containing versus non-nitrogen-containing bisphosphonate, use of oral bisphosphates should be considered the initial pharmacologic therapy for most postmenopausal women at high risk for fracture or when diagnosed with osteoporosis as well as in men in whom testosterone therapy is not indicated. Oral bisphosphates are preferred due to their efficacy, cost, and long-term safety data, but intravenous (IV) therapy should be used if oral bisphosphonate therapy is contraindicated, such as in patients with esophageal disorders or those with an inability to follow dosing requirements (eg, stay upright for 30 minutes). Serial BMD measurements are used to monitor treatment response. A positive response occurs when serial BMD measurements show stability or improvement.

Atypical subtrochanteric and femoral stress fractures are rare complications of chronic bisphosphonate therapy.[88–93] The orthopedic surgeon should have a high index of suspicion in the presence of thigh or hip pain and the "dreaded black line" in patients on bisphosphonate therapy, as they have an increased risk for complete stress fractures. These fractures are likely the result of propagated stress fracture whose repair is retarded by reduced osteoclast activity (**Fig. 3**) and impaired repair of microdamage due to prolonged bisphosphonate use.[91,92] The characteristic pattern is a low-energy fracture of the subtrochanteric region or femoral shaft with a simple, transverse pattern and hypertrophy of the diaphyseal cortex (**Fig. 4**).

There is lack of consensus regarding use of bisphosphonates following fractures. Animal models have shown that bisphosphonate therapy delays fracture healing both histologically and radiographically and alters the biomechanics of the healing callus.[94,95] The clinical studies and meta-analyses of perifracture bisphosphonate use in humans, however, have not shown similar detrimental effects of bisphosphonate initiation or continued use after sustaining an osteoporotic fracture.[96–100] Thus, bisphosphonates may have a use in the early postfragility fracture period, but there is not universal agreement that it is beneficial.

Teriparatide and denosumab

Teriparatide (FORTEO) is a recombinant active peptide of PTH and is the only anabolic agent used in the treatment of osteoporosis.[101] Denosumab (Prolia, Xgeva), a monoclonal antibody against RANK-L, prevents osteoclast maturation, thereby preventing breakdown of bone. In a randomized trial, combined teriparatide and denosumab increased BMD more than either agent alone and more than has been reported with

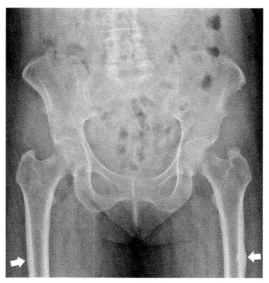

Fig. 3. AP pelvis radiograph of a 71-year-old woman with early insufficiency fractures in the setting of prolonged bisphosphonate use. Arrows highlight bilateral subtrochanteric diaphyseal cortical hypertrophic lesions. The patient received a total of 8 years of alendronate therapy with a 1-year bone holiday after the first 5 years.

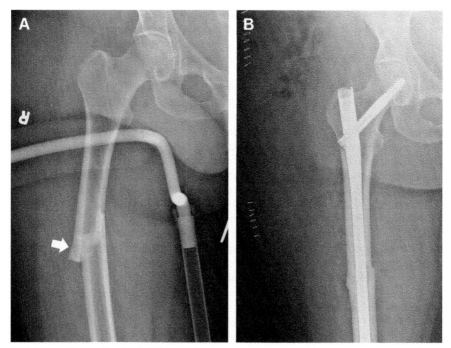

Fig. 4. AP radiograph of a left femur demonstrating a low-energy fracture of the femoral shaft with a simple, transverse pattern and hypertrophy of the diaphyseal cortex (*arrow*) (*A*), and postoperatively demonstrating interval placement of an intramedullary nail (*B*).

approved therapies.[102] Combination treatment using these agents might, therefore, be useful to treat patients at high risk of fracture.

PREOPERATIVE ASSESSMENT, OPTIMIZATION, AND CARE
Prioritization of Surgical Indications and Timing

Orthopedic procedures can classified into 3 general categories: elective, necessary, and emergent.[103] The general workup, assessment, and optimization of the geriatric orthopedic patient will significantly differ based on the urgency of the patient's surgery.

Elective surgeries are those that can be delayed without negative consequence to the patient. Necessary procedures are required in order to preserve the quality of life or decrease the risk of continued morbidity and are not truly life or limb threatening; it is within this category whereby controversy occasionally occurs between medical consultants and treating surgeons. In cases of geriatric trauma, expeditious care leads to improved outcomes and decreased morbidity and mortality. Thus, communication between all members of the medical and surgical teams is vital. Finally, surgeries considered emergent are either life or limb threatening; this category also includes procedures whereby severe compromise to the affected limb may occur if surgical intervention is not undertaken expeditiously. In many cases, emergent procedures are oftentimes performed before thorough medical evaluation and optimization because it is in the patient's best interest. It is therefore imperative in the evaluation of a geriatric orthopedic patient to determine: the category of procedure (emergent, urgent, or elective); the optimal time frame for surgical intervention; duration of the procedure; potentials for nonoperative management; and priority relative to other surgical cases. The extent of medical evaluation and further workup or workups is critically dependent on the surgical priority.

Preoperative Assessment and Evaluation

The authors recommend primary care physicians and/or geriatricians preoperatively evaluate patients physiologically 65 years and older, and all patients 80 years and older before surgery. The need for further evaluation by a cardiologist, with or without additional cardiac testing, should be determined by the primary care physician, geriatrician, and/or by the treating surgeons if any concerns remain. The purpose of this evaluation is not to "clear" a patient for surgery per se, as this may incorrectly imply that the procedure carries no risk for the patient. Rather, the goals of this evaluation are to identify pertinent medical problems, anticipate potential perioperative problems, assess the patient's risk and need for further interventions, and communicate these findings with the treating surgical team and anesthesiologist.

General laboratory medicine

Routine preoperative laboratory testing is not always needed. Specific testing should be based on a combination of patient factors and procedure risks. For the geriatric orthopedic patient undergoing intermediate- to high-risk surgery (arthroplasty, spine, trauma), it is recommended to order electrolytes, renal function, complete blood count (CBC), and hemostasis evaluation (eg, international normalized ratio). Optional tests, which should be considered in patients with certain comorbidities or in effort to further optimize the patient preoperatively, include liver function tests, albumin, prealbumin, blood glucose, and hemoglobin A1c. These tests are discussed later with indications for their use in specific patients.

The preoperative assessment

The perioperative consultation and preoperative assessment should focus on the issues relevant to the current surgery. These immediate concerns must be evaluated in terms of their severity, the planned surgical procedure, the patient's perioperative risk, and the need for further testing or intervention. Any other medical issues may be addressed after surgery or during subsequent outpatient visits. The following sections briefly touch on the factors to be considered in the preoperative evaluation (**Table 1**).

Cardiac Cardiovascular disease, including peripheral artery disease, predisposes patients to elevated risks of perioperative complications. The incidence of an adverse cardiovascular outcome in orthopedic surgery is related to the baseline risk. Use of risk calculators and functional metabolic equivalents (MET) should be used to determine need for further testing in cases of nonemergent surgery. Emergent cases should be allowed to proceed with risk stratification alone. If further testing in patients with poor or unknown functional capacity (<4 METs) will alter perioperative care or impact decision making, testing and treatment are recommended. Surgical management can be recommended if a patient is low risk or has moderate or better functional capacity (≥4 METs).

The general patient assessment should evaluate for ischemia, revascularization procedures, presence of atrial fibrillation, congestive heart failure, valvular heart disease, and peripheral artery disease as well as the medications used in management of these conditions. Very high-risk patients should be optimally treated before surgery. These patients include those with a recent myocardial infarction (≤60 days) or unstable angina, decompensated heart failure, high-grade arrhythmias, or hemodynamically important valvular heart disease.[104]

In cases of emergent surgery, the benefit of proceeding with surgery tends to outweigh the risk of waiting to perform additional testing and treatment. At-risk patients should be monitored and treated when necessary for possible cardiovascular complications postoperatively.

A preoperative electrocardiogram (ECG) should be ordered in all geriatric orthopedic patients. This baseline ECG should be evaluated for pathology and serves as a baseline ECG should abnormal changes occur postoperatively.

Pulmonary A significant cause of perioperative morbidity and mortality stems from pulmonary complications occurring postoperatively, underscoring the need for a thorough preoperative assessment. The most important tools for preoperative risk assessment include a careful history and physical examination. The preoperative physical

Table 1	
Factors to be considered in the preoperative evaluation	
Organ System	**Considerations**
Cardiac	Ischemia, revascularization, stents, atrial fibrillation, medications (beta-blockers, antihypertensives, rate/rhythm agents), congestive heart failure, peripheral artery disease, valvular disease
Pulmonary	COPD, smoking status, and history
Renal	Acute and/or chronic renal failure, urinary retention
Gastrointestinal	Nutrition, peptic ulcer disease, obesity, liver disease
Hematologic	Bleeding, clotting, anticoagulation
Endocrine	Diabetes, thyroid dysfunction

examination should be focused on evidence toward any degree of obstructive lung disease.[105] Careful attention should be given to patients with histories suggesting unrecognized chronic lung disease or heart failure, such as exercise intolerance, unexplained dyspnea, or cough. A systematic review by the American College of Physicians[106] grouped risk factors for perioperative pulmonary complications into patient-related and procedure-related risks. Patient-related risks factors include advanced age, American Society of Anesthesiologists class 2 or higher, functional dependence, chronic obstructive pulmonary disease (COPD), congestive heart failure, and metabolic and nutritional factors. Orthopedic-specific procedure-related risk factors include spine surgery, emergent surgery, use of general anesthesia, vascular surgery, and prolonged surgery.

Routine preoperative chest radiographs in healthy asymptomatic patients rarely change preoperative management.[107] Ambulatory procedures, in particular, may not benefit from preoperative chest radiographs.[108] However, chest radiographs can be reasonably obtained preoperatively in patients with known cardiopulmonary disease, smokers, and those with multiple risk factors.

Renal Renal function should, in general, always be assessed in geriatric patients undergoing orthopedic surgery. Although mild to moderate renal impairment is usually asymptomatic, the degree of impairment as well as its prevalence increases with age. Large intraoperative blood loss and postoperative third spacing of fluids can cause acute kidney injury and can exacerbate chronic renal failure. The presence of renal insufficiency is also an independent risk factor for postoperative pulmonary complications.[106] Chronic kidney disease is an independent risk factor of postoperative death and cardiovascular events with similar strength of association to diabetes, stroke, and coronary disease[109]; within the orthopedic literature it has been identified as a predictor of postoperative mortality associated with a univariate acute mortality of 9%.[110] Patients with chronic kidney disease, in particular, have mortalities of 45% within 2 years of sustaining a hip fracture.[111]

In addition, certain narcotic pain medications and muscle relaxants should have their dosages adjusted or should be avoided in patients with compromised kidney function when they are metabolized renally.

Gastrointestinal and nutrition The preoperative laboratory evaluation of nutritional status, which is generally used to assess wound healing potential as well as mortality, includes prealbumin, C-reactive protein (CRP), albumin, and total lymphocyte count (TLC). These laboratory markers should be optimized (albumin >3.5, TLC >1500 cell/mm^3) before and within the perioperative period if possible. Malnourishment, within older persons, is an independent risk factor for all-cause mortality[112] and can identify patients with greater risk of readmission.[113] In addition, malnutrition is associated with worse functional status with more frequent remaining functional loss.[114] If a patient is hospitalized, and their surgery delayed, it is important to avoid disruptions of nutritional intake due to persistent NPO status.

Acute-phase proteins, for example, CRP, are synthesized during hyperinflammatory states at the expense of prealbumin. For this reason, prealbumin may not be a sensitive marker for evaluating the adequacy of nutritional support in critically ill patients[115]; with low CRP levels, prealbumin may be used to assess acute protein status and monitor the response to nutritional support.[115,116]

Liver function screening tests are not warranted in asymptotic patients because they are almost always unhelpful in predicting outcomes and not necessary in optimizing surgical outcomes.[117]

Box 2
Preoperative assessment and optimization pearls

Preprocedure cardiologic intervention should be performed, if deemed necessary, to minimize perioperative surgical risk of orthopedic procedures

Unrecognized cardiopulmonary dysfunction, specifically, restrictive lung disease, significantly contributes to postoperative pulmonary complications

Chronic kidney disease contributes toward higher mortalities in patients undergoing orthopedic procedures

Postoperative medication (narcotics, muscle relaxants) dose adjustments are necessary in patients with compromised renal function

Nutrition status should be optimized in the perioperative period to decrease complications

Obesity leads to nearly universally poorer orthopedic outcomes

Oral vitamin K facilitates a hepatic first pass effect when compared with subcutaneous or IV administration

Coagulopathies are exacerbated by consumptive coagulopathies occurring with fractures

Blood glucose optimization improves wound healing and decreases infection

---

Obesity causes significant perioperative issues for orthopedic surgery, including difficulty positioning, higher infection rates, higher rates of thromboembolism, increased loads across implants causing premature and early failures, increased postoperative pain, impaired postoperative mobility, and worse patient outcomes.[118–121] Despite these clear perioperative risks, there is little that can be done acutely to improve outcomes, so it is uncertain whether the preoperative approach to obese patients should differ from the general population.[122]

Hematologic Patients receiving chronic anticoagulation should have this discontinued shortly before surgery and resumed once risk of bleeding is minimized, generally within one to 2 days after surgery. Patients who are coagulopathic and require urgent or emergent surgery should receive vitamin K and/or fresh frozen plasma to correct the coagulopathy. Oral forms of vitamin K are advantageous over IV and subcutaneous injections because they allow for first pass through the liver where coagulation factors are synthesized. It should be noted that bleeding from a fracture will exacerbate the coagulopathy through utilization of a considerable amount of coagulation factors (consumptive coagulopathy), so discontinuation of the anticoagulant medication without concomitant administration of vitamin K or fresh frozen plasma may be associated with worsening of the anticoagulation (**Box 2**).

Comanagement

Comanagement, whereby the surgery and medicine services share responsibility for the patient, has become increasingly popular in geriatric orthopedic surgery in the last decade, especially for patients with hip fractures. More recently, the concept of comanagement is being used increasingly in geriatric patients undergoing elective procedures, specifically for patients undergoing total hip and total knee arthroplasty. Rates of comanagement are also increasing for patients undergoing urgent and emergent procedures. The benefits of comanagement are numerous. Patients evaluated preoperatively by a geriatric team were more likely to return home following surgery than were patients first seen postoperatively.[123] Comanagement within orthopedics results in decreased complications and length of stay[124,125]; similar benefits are also seen across a broad spectrum of different surgeries.[126] Rehospitalization rates have also been shown to decrease with use of geriatric comanagement.[127] Finally, satisfaction among clinicians on each service is high with comanagement models.[128] The authors therefore recommend formal comanagement implementation and use, modified as needed to a particular medical center, whenever possible for orthopedic patients.

The Orthopedic Evaluation

When assessing the geriatric patient for surgery, the orthopedic surgeon must be cognizant of the indications and goals of surgery.

In general, the orthopedic surgeon should consider the following when assessing the risks and benefits of surgery: early motion/mobility, capacity to heal, presence of multiple fractures, fracture alignment, ultimate function, comfort, and pain relief. It is important to mobilize the geriatric patient as early as possible. By weighing each consideration, the decision of whether to proceed with surgery, and which surgical procedure is best, usually becomes apparent. Ultimately, the goal of any orthopedic surgical procedure is to allow for early mobility and maximal recovery of function, while avoiding perioperative complications, infection, and healing complications.

The recovery from orthopedic procedures will, at least temporarily, cause a decrease in functional level, resulting in loss of independence. Preoperative predictors of home discharges are correlated with age, cognitive ability, and number of comorbidities. The medical and surgical gestalt of the patient combined with an assessment of their social factors is useful in guiding discharge disposition. Patients discharged to subacute nursing facilities and postacute care rehabilitation centers have significantly higher chance of hospital readmission within 90 days of surgery.[129] Moreover, rehabilitation facility charges are the most significant driver of cost in the postacute care phase,[130] with cost increases up to 30% reported when compared with patients who are sent home.[131] Therefore, significant efforts should be put forth by the patient, the patient's support and the health care team with regards to intensive pre operative and perioperative optimization for home discharges, and identification patients at risk of needing postacute care to allow for expeditious disposition planning in the immediate postoperative period.

OPERATIVE AND INTRAOPERATIVE CONSIDERATIONS
Preoperative Planning

The preoperative plan for geriatric orthopedic surgery significantly differs from the plan for younger patients due to the need for early mobilization, the phenotypic differences in bone quality secondary to aging, the differences in soft tissue quality, previous surgeries, and the functional demands placed on the implants.

The goal of major elective orthopedic procedures in the geriatric patient is improved mobility as a byproduct of decreased pain (eg, arthroplasty, spinal decompression). Geriatric fracture care, more than elective procedures, embodies the need for early mobility and retention of functional status. The disability generated due to a fracture should be optimally addressed to allow for early rehabilitation directed at the impairment, and retention of functional status, including activities of daily living (ADLs). It is for this reason the authors recommend preoperative planning aimed at maximizing the ability to bear weight in the postoperative period using supplemental fixation (longer plates, more screws, use of cables, and so forth). In many cases, joint replacing procedures should be considered over open reduction internal fixation to facilitate early postoperative functional gains.

Osteoporosis and osteopenia often will have a dramatic impact how orthopedic implants are used. Geriatric patients with implants often require stronger fixation in order to allow for earlier weight bearing. Low-energy geriatric fractures often present with significant comminution. Cautious use of methylmethacrylate cement augmentation of bone can be used to fill large bony voids, improve fixation strength, reduce implant failure, and allow for earlier weight bearing.

Malnutrition and nutritional compromise are common in geriatric patients. As previously stated, nutritional status should be optimized when possible during the perioperative period. Minimally invasive procedures (**Figs. 5** and **6**), including indirect reduction techniques, minimal soft tissue dissection, and minimal devitalization of the bone due to exposure, improve healing potential. Therefore, intramedullary devices (ie, intramedullary nails) should be used, when possible, in the treatment of geriatric fractures.

The possibility of previous surgeries and orthopedic implants (eg, arthroplasty) emphasizes the need for complete radiographic imaging, which includes the bone or bones to be operated on and the joints above and below said bone. If previous hardware is seen, detailed operative reports should be obtained when possible to plan for the availability of the correct instruments in the operating room at the time of orthopedic implantation. The presence of previous implants can necessitate alternative surgical plans and staging of procedures. If a referral is made for an elective surgical case, the surgeon must attempt to obtain and include all previous operative reports.

Geriatric patients are, in general, lower-demand individuals. However, mobility is vital to the geriatric patient because inactivity is significantly associated with increased morbidity and mortality. Fractures, which may be managed nonoperatively in younger patients, are often treated with surgery to optimize early mobility, range of motion, and functional independence.

Intraoperative Considerations

Anticoagulation is especially important in the geriatric orthopedic patient. Although only 1.5% to 2% of the population in developed countries have atrial fibrillation,

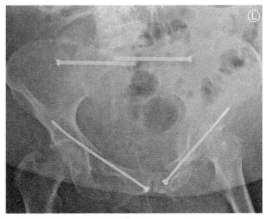

Fig. 5. AP pelvis demonstrating minimally invasive, percutaneous fixation of the pelvic ring including bilateral superior pubic rami, right and left sacral fractures in an osteoporotic trauma patient with multiple medical comorbidities.

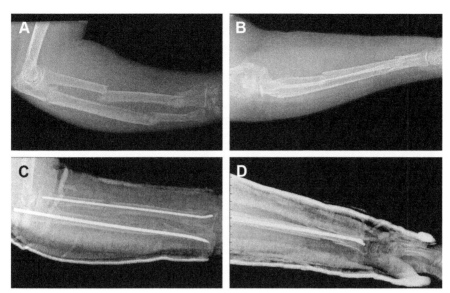

Fig. 6. AP (A) and lateral (B) radiographs of a right forearm demonstrating comminuted, segmental fractures of the radius and ulna. Postoperative AP (C) and lateral (D) radiographs demonstrate intramedullary fixation of the radius and ulna. Intramedullary fixation with indirect reduction techniques was selected to minimize soft tissue dissection and devitalization of the bone allowing for improved healing potential.

10% of patients older than the age of 80 are affected, and there is an exponential increase in the very elderly, which largely drives anticoagulant use.[132] Preoperative anticoagulation status and plans for future anticoagulation should be evaluated with the anesthesiologist to assist with determining optimal anesthesia care. Anticoagulated patients should not receive central neuraxial blocks. Peripheral nerve blockade, however, may provide an alternative in these patients, excluding lumbar plexus blocks. If a patient is to receive a neuraxial block, low molecular weight heparin should not be administered within 12 hours of the neuraxial block. A recent study in hip fracture patients[133] found the use of general anesthesia and conversion from regional to general anesthesia to be associated with higher mortality risk during in-hospital stay compared with regional anesthetic techniques. They also found general anesthesia to be associated with a higher risk of all-cause readmission compared with regional anesthesia. Therefore, although regional anesthesia is recommended when possible, careful patient selection remains critical.

Elderly patients have less physiologic reserve to tolerate hemorrhage. Several major orthopedic surgeries have the potential to result in significant blood loss and the need for perioperative and postoperative allogenic blood transfusions. The management of surgical blood loss has evolved alongside modern surgery, and widespread conservation strategies have been implemented. Intraoperative management includes controlled hypotensive anesthesia, use of tourniquets when indicated, cell salvage techniques, and use of tranexamic acid. Controlled hypotensive anesthesia assists the surgeon with visualization, limits intraoperative blood loss, and may even decrease deep vein thrombosis by limiting consumption of anticoagulants like antithrombin III and hemodilution that occurs during surgical blood loss.

Finally, bone cement implantation syndrome (BCIS) is a rare form of intraoperative pulmonary embolism characterized by hypotension and hypoxemia, involving pressurized bone cement within orthopedic surgery. The syndrome is most often seen in cemented hemiarthroplasty in osteoporotic geriatric patients, but also occurs in total hip and total knee replacement surgeries[134] and has a huge impact on early and late mortality. BCIS is treated supportively with hydration, 100% inspired oxygen, and vasopressors if necessary.[134–136] The incidence of BCIS may be lessened by advance notification of the anesthesiologist that cement will be used, and by waiting until the cement is thickened or "doughy" before insertion within the bone.

POSTOPERATIVE CARE
Postoperative Evaluation

Similar to the preoperative evaluation wherein a complete assessment of the patient and their comorbidities is required, monitoring and evaluation of patients' comorbid risks as well as inherent risks of surgery should be performed throughout the postoperative period. Early mobility is a key driver in decreasing risk of many postoperative complications. The following sections touch on care in the immediate postoperative period.

Mobility
Early mobility in the postoperative period cannot be emphasized enough. Postoperative weight bearing should be maximized when possible. Early range of motion should be encouraged, but may not be possible due to splinting of the operative extremity. Evaluation with physical and occupational therapy services should be used to assist with gait training, weight bearing on the operative extremity, and reducing disability. Liberal consultation with physical therapy (PT) should be undertaken to encourage patient mobility.

Nursing staff also plays a significant role in the postoperative mobility of geriatric patients by maximizing their time spent out of bed (eg, sitting in a chair, using a commode vs bedpan). Improving and maximizing mobility decreases ultimate disability and has the potential to reduce postoperative complications.

Pressure-induced skin and soft tissue injuries are among the most common conditions encountered in hospitalized patients and in those requiring long-term care.[137] Geriatric patients should be repositioned at least every 2 hours to relieve tissue pressure. Turning and positioning techniques should minimize friction and shear forces.[138] Screening should occur formally during nursing assessments and be reported to the treating team, when noted. Further optimizing nutritional status limits propagation of soft tissue injury and optimizes healing. A team approach involving the clinical staff, patients, and families is essential to reduce the development of pressure sores.

Cardiopulmonary
Pulmonary complications are a major cause of morbidity and mortality during the postoperative period and exist on a spectrum from atelectasis to spontaneous death due to pulmonary venous thromboembolism. Deep breathing and incentive spirometry should be recommended to geriatric patients with comorbid pulmonary disease undergoing orthopedic surgery to reduce postoperative pulmonary complications. Early mobilization after orthopedic surgery facilitates deep breathing and also reduces the risk of deep venous thrombosis.

Venous thromboembolism is a devastating complication and occurs from loss of anticoagulants (eg, antithrombin III) by consumption and hemodilution during surgical blood loss. Venous stasis, which promotes thrombosis, may result from manipulation of the operative extremity, tourniquet use, and hypothermia resulting in vasoconstriction.[139] Prophylactic anticoagulation substantially reduces the risk of venous thromboembolism in patients undergoing orthopedic surgery. The American Academy of Orthopaedic Surgeons recommends using pharmacologic agents and/or mechanical compressive devices for the prevention of venous thromboembolism in patients undergoing elective hip or knee arthroplasty, and who are not at elevated risk beyond that of the surgery itself for venous thromboembolism or bleeding.[140] Consensus regarding the use and duration of prophylactic anticoagulation should be determined by the procedure, patient risk factors, and discussion between the medical and surgical teams.

Gastrointestinal
Geriatric patients should be regularly screened to ensure passing of flatus and regularity of bowel movements. Narcotic use reduces peristalsis through binding of specific receptors in the gastrointestinal tract and central nervous system contributing to postoperative constipation and long-term obstipation. Prophylactic use of contact cathartic (eg, senna), stool softeners, and osmotic laxatives (eg, polyethylene glycol) should be considered in all patients actively taking narcotic pain medication to limit potential complications.

Postoperative paralytic ileus is a benign condition that usually resolves without serious sequelae. In the presence of prolonged postoperative ileus, or should concern develop, the ileus should be evaluated to exclude other causes of ileus and/or postoperative abdominal distension. The evaluation should include plain radiography and laboratory studies: electrolyte panel, including magnesium, blood urea nitrogen, CBC, liver function tests, amylase and lipase.

Wound healing
The potential for wound healing should be optimized in the perioperative and postoperative period. All patient risk factors should be addressed. Generalizable risk factors include obesity, diabetes, nicotine use, and malnutrition. Consultation with nutritionists for dietary modification and protein supplementation recommendations should be considered in patients with metabolic syndromes, obesity, and diabetes. Smoking cessation counseling should be provided to every patient. Nicotine replacement (ie, gum, patches) should be limited when possible, especially if wound-healing concerns arise.

POSTHOSPITAL CARE
Rehabilitation

Geriatric surgical patients may be disabled by acute and/or chronic health issues, and personal and environmental factors. Surgical and medical interventions target physical health issues, whereas rehabilitation interventions are designed to address all the covariates impacting the patient's well-being.[141] Thus, it is important to make recommendations after assessing the patient's functional and social status.

Involvement of PT and occupational therapy is a necessary component of hospital discharge planning. Early involvement of therapists becomes increasingly necessary in geriatric patients for whom there is concern about the ability to return home due to limitations in self-care or mobility. The most appropriate rehabilitation strategies need to be based on the specific cause of functional impairment. Postacute rehabilitation facilities serve as intermediary centers, allowing geriatric patients to be discharged from the hospital, but continue to have sufficient support in their ADLs and instrumental ADLs. However, research has shown orthopedic patients discharged to postacute rehabilitation have a significantly higher chance of hospital readmission within 90 days of surgery,[129] which is likely a function of lower baseline functional status, and less physiologic and physical reserve.

Functional home exercise regimens are also appropriate for many geriatric patients as their ADLs will dictate the demands of therapy. Specific guidelines and protocols are lacking if a more formal therapy program is to be undertaken. Early and frequent PT has been shown to improve outcomes.[142] Although extended duration PT was found to maximize functional outcomes in hip fracture patients,[143,144] limited therapy may be appropriate when therapy has restored functional demands. Finally, patients undergoing elective arthroplasty procedures may benefit from participation in "prehab" therapy.[145,146]

Postoperative Clinic

The postoperative clinic visit for geriatric patients presents unique social challenges. Often, practical considerations getting patients to clinic are created as a result of compromised functional status. Formal medical transportation must oftentimes be arranged if friends or family members are not available. When patients return to clinic from skilled nursing or residential facilities, a caregiver or certified patient assistant usually accompanies them, displacing them from the facility. For these reasons, patients should be discharged home when possible to avoid the burdensome requirements surrounding transportation. In addition, the number of extraneous clinic visits should be limited when possible.

The postoperative clinic visit allows the orthopedic surgeon to monitor the area or areas of interest for healing and assess the patient's perception of functional improvements. Radiographs provide an assessment of union, implant and construct position and stability, and are used to monitor for complications.

Assessment of Outcomes

Patient-reported outcomes should be collected at every patient visit following any surgical procedure. PROMIS (Patient-Reported Outcomes Measurement Information System) is a set of person-centered measures that evaluates and monitors physical, mental, and social health. PROMIS has been validated across a large number of orthopedic patient populations and surgical procedures. Collecting and trending PROMIS scores is recommended for monitoring outcomes.

Radiographic outcomes should also be assessed during each patient visit. Week-to-week and month-to-month changes are often subtle, going unnoticed. Thus, radiographs should be scrutinized for subtle changes from the previous visit, and against the earliest postoperative radiographs. Bony remodeling and healing should be evaluated. Scrutinize and assess the bone or bones for adequate and timely healing as increasing comorbidities and vitamin D deficiencies may reduce healing potential. If nonoperative treatment was elected, weight bearing should commence and be advanced when possible to limit functional losses.

REFERENCES

1. Ortman JM, Velkoff VA, Hogan H. An aging nation: the older population in the United States. Population estimates and projections. US Census Bureau; 2012. Available at: https://www.census.gov/prod/2014pubs/p25-1140.pdf. Accessed October 5, 2018.

2. United Nations Department of Economic and Social Affairs Population Division. World population ageing: 1950–2050. Available at: http://www.un.org/esa/population/publications/worldageing19502050/. Accessed February 10, 2018.

3. Wright NC, Looker AC, Saag KG, et al. The recent prevalence of osteoporosis and low bone mass in the United States based on bone mineral density at the femoral neck or lumbar spine. J Bone Miner Res 2014;29(11):2520–6.

4. Bone health and osteoporosis: A report of the Surgeon General. Rockville (MD): Office of the Surgeon General; 2004.

5. Gardner MJ, Flik KR, Mooar P, et al. Improvement in the undertreatment of osteoporosis following hip fracture. J Bone Joint Surg Am 2002;84-A(8):1342–8.

6. Gardner MJ, Brophy RH, Demetrakopoulos D, et al. Interventions to improve osteoporosis treatment following hip fracture. A prospective, randomized trial. J Bone Joint Surg Am 2005;87(1):3–7.

7. Bahl S, Coates PS, Greenspan SL. The management of osteoporosis following hip fracture: have we improved our care? Osteoporos Int 2003;14(11):884–8.

8. Follin SL, Black JN, McDermott MT. Lack of diagnosis and treatment of osteoporosis in men and women after hip fracture. Pharmacotherapy 2003;23(2):190–8.

9. Harrington JT, Broy SB, Derosa AM, et al. Hip fracture patients are not treated for osteoporosis: a call to action. Arthritis Rheum 2002;47(6):651–4.

10. Kamel HK, Hussain MS, Tariq S, et al. Failure to diagnose and treat osteoporosis in elderly patients hospitalized with hip fracture. Am J Med 2000;109(4):326–8.

11. Morgan EN, Crawford DA, Scully WF, et al. Medical management of fragility fractures of the distal radius. Orthopedics 2014;37(12):e1068–73.

12. Queally JM, Kiernan C, Shaikh M, et al. Initiation of osteoporosis assessment in the fracture clinic results in improved osteoporosis management: a randomised controlled trial. Osteoporos Int 2013;24(3):1089–94.

13. Marshall D, Johnell O, Wedel H. Meta-analysis of how well measures of bone mineral density predict occurrence of osteoporotic fractures. BMJ 1996; 312(7041):1254–9.

14. Cummings SR, Bates D, Black DM. Clinical use of bone densitometry: scientific review. JAMA 2002;288(15):1889–97.

15. Siris ES, Chen YT, Abbott TA, et al. Bone mineral density thresholds for pharmacological intervention to prevent fractures. Arch Intern Med 2004;164(10): 1108–12.

16. Sornay-Rendu E, Munoz F, Garnero P, et al. Identification of osteopenic women at high risk of fracture: the OFELY study. J Bone Miner Res 2005;20(10):1813–9.

17. Schuit SC, van der Klift M, Weel AE, et al. Fracture incidence and association with bone mineral density in elderly men and women: the Rotterdam Study. Bone 2004;34(1):195–202.

18. Kanis JA. Diagnosis of osteoporosis and assessment of fracture risk. Lancet 2002;359(9321):1929–36.

19. Kanis JA, Johnell O, Oden A, et al. FRAX and the assessment of fracture probability in men and women from the UK. Osteoporos Int 2008;19(4):385–97.

20. Kanis JA, Johnell O, De Laet C, et al. A meta-analysis of previous fracture and subsequent fracture risk. Bone 2004;35(2):375–82.

21. Kanis JA, Oden A, Johnell O, et al. The use of clinical risk factors enhances the performance of BMD in the prediction of hip and osteoporotic fractures in men and women. Osteoporos Int 2007;18(8):1033–46.

22. Dawson-Hughes B, Tosteson AN, Melton LJ 3rd, et al. Implications of absolute fracture risk assessment for osteoporosis practice guidelines in the USA. Osteoporos Int 2008;19(4):449–58.

23. Vaidya R, Kubiak EN, Bergin PF, et al. Complications of anterior subcutaneous internal fixation for unstable pelvis fractures: a multicenter study. Clin Orthop Relat Res 2012;470(8):2124–31.

24. Burge R, Dawson-Hughes B, Solomon DH, et al. Incidence and economic burden of osteoporosis-related fractures in the United States, 2005-2025. J Bone Miner Res 2007;22(3):465–75.

25. Balasubramanian A, Tosi LL, Lane JM, et al. Declining rates of osteoporosis management following fragility fractures in the U.S., 2000 through 2009. J Bone Joint Surg Am 2014;96(7):e52.

26. Ganda K, Puech M, Chen JS, et al. Models of care for the secondary prevention of osteoporotic fractures: a systematic review and meta-analysis. Osteoporos Int 2013;24(2):393–406.

27. Newman ED, Ayoub WT, Starkey RH, et al. Osteoporosis disease management in a rural health care population: hip fracture reduction and reduced costs in postmenopausal women after 5 years. Osteoporos Int 2003;14(2):146–51.

28. McLellan AR, Gallacher SJ, Fraser M, et al. The fracture liaison service: success of a program for the evaluation and management of patients with osteoporotic fracture. Osteoporos Int 2003;14(12):1028–34.

29. Dell R, Greene D, Schelkun SR, et al. Osteoporosis disease management: the role of the orthopaedic surgeon. J Bone Joint Surg Am 2008;90(Suppl 4): 188–94.

30. Harrington JT, Deal CL. Successes and failures in improving osteoporosis care after fragility fracture: results of a multiple-site clinical improvement project. Arthritis Rheum 2006;55(5):724–8.

31. Edwards BJ, Bunta AD, Simonelli C, et al. Prior fractures are common in patients with subsequent hip fractures. Clin Orthop Relat Res 2007;461:226–30.

32. Choma TJ, Rechtine GR, McGuire RA Jr, et al. Treating the aging Spine. J Am Acad Orthop Surg 2015;23(12):e91–100.

33. Caruso G, Milani L, Marko T, et al. Surgical treatment of periprosthetic femoral fractures: a retrospective study with functional and radiological outcomes from 2010 to 2016. Eur J Orthop Surg Traumatol 2018;28(5):931–8.

34. Forster MC, Komarsamy B, Davison JN. Distal femoral fractures: a review of fixation methods. Injury 2006;37(2):97–108.

35. Oyen J, Brudvik C, Gjesdal CG, et al. Osteoporosis as a risk factor for distal radial fractures: a case-control study. J Bone Joint Surg Am 2011;93(4):348–56.

36. Levin LS, Rozell JC, Pulos N. Distal radius fractures in the elderly. J Am Acad Orthop Surg 2017;25(3):179–87.

37. Mehling I, Hessmann MH, Rommens PM. Stabilization of fatigue fractures of the dorsal pelvis with a trans-sacral bar. Operative technique and outcome. Injury 2012;43(4):446–51.

38. Zhuang XM, Yu BS, Zheng ZM, et al. Effect of the degree of osteoporosis on the biomechanical anchoring strength of the sacral pedicle screws: an in vitro comparison between unaugmented bicortical screws and polymethylmethacrylate augmented unicortical screws. Spine (Phila Pa 1976) 2010;35(19):E925–31.

39. Prieto-Alhambra D, Javaid MK, Judge A, et al. Fracture risk before and after total hip replacement in patients with osteoarthritis: potential benefits of bisphosphonate use. Arthritis Rheum 2011;63(4):992–1001.

40. Makela KT, Eskelinen A, Pulkkinen P, et al. Total hip arthroplasty for primary osteoarthritis in patients fifty-five years of age or older. An analysis of the Finnish arthroplasty registry. J Bone Joint Surg Am 2008;90(10):2160–70.

41. Fitzpatrick SK, Casemyr NE, Zurakowski D, et al. The effect of osteoporosis on outcomes of operatively treated distal radius fractures. J Hand Surg Am 2012; 37(10):2027–34.
42. Grant KD, Busse EC, Park DK, et al. Internal fixation of osteoporotic bone. J Am Acad Orthop Surg 2018;26(5):166–74.
43. Rothberg DL, Lee MA. Internal fixation of osteoporotic fractures. Curr Osteoporos Rep 2015;13(1):16–21.
44. Stadelmann VA, Bretton E, Terrier A, et al. Calcium phosphate cement augmentation of cancellous bone screws can compensate for the absence of cortical fixation. J Biomech 2010;43(15):2869–74.
45. Dell RM, Greene D, Anderson D, et al. Osteoporosis disease management: what every orthopaedic surgeon should know. J Bone Joint Surg Am 2009;91(Suppl 6):79–86.
46. Norman AW. From vitamin D to hormone D: fundamentals of the vitamin D endocrine system essential for good health. Am J Clin Nutr 2008;88(2):491S–9S.
47. Mithal A, Wahl DA, Bonjour JP, et al. Global vitamin D status and determinants of hypovitaminosis D. Osteoporos Int 2009;20(11):1807–20.
48. Yetley EA. Assessing the vitamin D status of the US population. Am J Clin Nutr 2008;88(2):558S–64S.
49. Holick MF. Vitamin D deficiency. N Engl J Med 2007;357(3):266–81.
50. Lee RH, Weber T, Colon-Emeric C. Comparison of cost-effectiveness of vitamin D screening with that of universal supplementation in preventing falls in community-dwelling older adults. J Am Geriatr Soc 2013;61(5):707–14.
51. Centers for Medicare & Medicaid Services, Division of Quality, Evaluation and Health Outcomes. Quality measures compendium: medicaid and SCHIP quality improvement, vol. 2.0. U.S. Department of Commerce - National Technical Reports Library; 2007.
52. Lavernia CJ, Villa JM, Iacobelli DA, et al. Vitamin D insufficiency in patients with THA: prevalence and effects on outcome. Clin Orthop Relat Res 2014;472(2): 681–6.
53. Andres BA, Childs BR, Vallier HA. Treatment of hypovitaminosis D in an orthopaedic trauma population. J Orthop Trauma 2018;32(4):e129–33.
54. Quraishi SA, Bittner EA, Blum L, et al. Association between preoperative 25-hydroxyvitamin D level and hospital-acquired infections following Roux-en-Y gastric bypass surgery. JAMA Surg 2014;149(2):112–8.
55. Holick MF, Binkley NC, Bischoff-Ferrari HA, et al. Evaluation, treatment, and prevention of vitamin D deficiency: an Endocrine Society clinical practice guideline. J Clin Endocrinol Metab 2011;96(7):1911–30.
56. Sanders KM, Stuart AL, Williamson EJ, et al. Annual high-dose oral vitamin D and falls and fractures in older women: a randomized controlled trial. JAMA 2010;303(18):1815–22.
57. Ross AC, Manson JE, Abrams SA, et al. The 2011 report on dietary reference intakes for calcium and vitamin D from the Institute of Medicine: what clinicians need to know. J Clin Endocrinol Metab 2011;96(1):53–8.
58. Vieth R. Vitamin D supplementation, 25-hydroxyvitamin D concentrations, and safety. Am J Clin Nutr 1999;69(5):842–56.
59. Vieth R. Vitamin D and cancer mini-symposium: the risk of additional vitamin D. Ann Epidemiol 2009;19(7):441–5.
60. Mirza F, Canalis E. Management of endocrine disease: secondary osteoporosis: pathophysiology and management. Eur J Endocrinol 2015;173(3):R131–51.

61. Bailey RL, Dodd KW, Goldman JA, et al. Estimation of total usual calcium and vitamin D intakes in the United States. J Nutr 2010;140(4):817–22.

62. Cranney A, Guyatt G, Griffith L, et al. Meta-analyses of therapies for postmeno-pausal osteoporosis. IX: summary of meta-analyses of therapies for postmeno-pausal osteoporosis. Endocr Rev 2002;23(4):570–8.

63. Silk LN, Greene DA, Baker MK. The effect of calcium or calcium and vitamin D supplementation on bone mineral density in healthy males: a systematic review and meta-analysis. Int J Sport Nutr Exerc Metab 2015;25(5):510–24.

64. Rozenberg S, Body JJ, Bruyere O, et al. Effects of dairy products consumption on health: benefits and beliefs–a commentary from the belgian bone club and the european society for clinical and economic aspects of osteoporosis, osteo-arthritis and musculoskeletal diseases. Calcif Tissue Int 2016;98(1):1–17.

65. Ethgen O, Hiligsmann M, Burlet N, et al. Cost-effectiveness of personalized sup-plementation with vitamin D-rich dairy products in the prevention of osteoporotic fractures. Osteoporos Int 2016;27(1):301–8.

66. Jackson RD, LaCroix AZ, Gass M, et al. Calcium plus vitamin D supplementation and the risk of fractures. N Engl J Med 2006;354(7):669–83.

67. Kim KM, Choi SH, Lim S, et al. Interactions between dietary calcium intake and bone mineral density or bone geometry in a low calcium intake population (KNHANES IV 2008-2010). J Clin Endocrinol Metab 2014;99(7):2409–17.

68. Daly RM, Brown M, Bass S, et al. Calcium- and vitamin D3-fortified milk reduces bone loss at clinically relevant skeletal sites in older men: a 2-year randomized controlled trial. J Bone Miner Res 2006;21(3):397–405.

69. Meier C, Woitge HW, Witte K, et al. Supplementation with oral vitamin D3 and calcium during winter prevents seasonal bone loss: a randomized controlled open-label prospective trial. J Bone Miner Res 2004;19(8):1221–30.

70. Reid IR, Ames RW, Evans MC, et al. Effect of calcium supplementation on bone loss in postmenopausal women. N Engl J Med 1993;328(7):460–4.

71. Dawson-Hughes B, Harris SS, Krall EA, et al. Effect of calcium and vitamin D supplementation on bone density in men and women 65 years of age or older. N Engl J Med 1997;337(10):670–6.

72. Reid IR, Mason B, Horne A, et al. Randomized controlled trial of calcium in healthy older women. Am J Med 2006;119(9):777–85.

73. Reid IR, Ames R, Mason B, et al. Randomized controlled trial of calcium sup-plementation in healthy, nonosteoporotic, older men. Arch Intern Med 2008; 168(20):2276–82.

74. Storm D, Eslin R, Porter ES, et al. Calcium supplementation prevents seasonal bone loss and changes in biochemical markers of bone turnover in elderly New England women: a randomized placebo-controlled trial. J Clin Endocrinol Metab 1998;83(11):3817–25.

75. Riggs BL, Wahner HW, Seeman E, et al. Changes in bone mineral density of the proximal femur and spine with aging. Differences between the postmenopausal and senile osteoporosis syndromes. J Clin Invest 1982;70(4):716–23.

76. Rizzoli R, Poser J, Burgi U. Nuclear thyroid hormone receptors in cultured bone cells. Metabolism 1986;35(1):71–4.

77. Abu EO, Bord S, Horner A, et al. The expression of thyroid hormone receptors in human bone. Bone 1997;21(2):137–42.

78. Sato K, Han DC, Fujii Y, et al. Thyroid hormone stimulates alkaline phosphatase activity in cultured rat osteoblastic cells (ROS 17/2.8) through 3,5,3'-triiodo-L-thyronine nuclear receptors. Endocrinology 1987;120(5):1873–81.

79. Mundy GR, Shapiro JL, Bandelin JG, et al. Direct stimulation of bone resorption by thyroid hormones. J Clin Invest 1976;58(3):529–34.
80. Britto JM, Fenton AJ, Holloway WR, et al. Osteoblasts mediate thyroid hormone stimulation of osteoclastic bone resorption. Endocrinology 1994;134(1):169–76.
81. Karsenty G, Bouchard P, Ulmann A, et al. Elevated metabolic clearance rate of 1 alpha,25-dihydroxyvitamin D3 in hyperthyroidism. Acta Endocrinol (Copenh) 1985;110(1):70–4.
82. Cosman F, de Beur SJ, LeBoff MS, et al. Clinician's guide to prevention and treatment of osteoporosis. Osteoporos Int 2014;25(10):2359–81.
83. Dawson-Hughes B, National Osteoporosis Foundation Guide Committee. A revised clinician's guide to the prevention and treatment of osteoporosis. J Clin Endocrinol Metab 2008;93(7):2463–5.
84. Dunford JE. Molecular targets of the nitrogen containing bisphosphonates: the molecular pharmacology of prenyl synthase inhibition. Curr Pharm Des 2010; 16(27):2961–9.
85. Russell RG. Bisphosphonates: mode of action and pharmacology. Pediatrics 2007;119(Suppl 2):S150–62.
86. Rogers MJ. From molds and macrophages to mevalonate: a decade of progress in understanding the molecular mode of action of bisphosphonates. Calcif Tissue Int 2004;75(6):451–61.
87. van beek E, Lowik C, van der Pluijm G, et al. The role of geranylgeranylation in bone resorption and its suppression by bisphosphonates in fetal bone explants in vitro: a clue to the mechanism of action of nitrogen-containing bisphosphonates. J Bone Miner Res 1999;14(5):722–9.
88. Adler RA, El-Hajj Fuleihan G, Bauer DC, et al. Managing osteoporosis in patients on long-term bisphosphonate treatment: report of a task force of the american society for bone and mineral research. J Bone Miner Res 2016;31(1):16–35.
89. Shane E, Burr D, Ebeling PR, et al. Atypical subtrochanteric and diaphyseal femoral fractures: report of a task force of the American Society for Bone and Mineral Research. J Bone Miner Res 2010;25(11):2267–94.
90. Shane E, Burr D, Abrahamsen B, et al. Atypical subtrochanteric and diaphyseal femoral fractures: second report of a task force of the American Society for Bone and Mineral Research. J Bone Miner Res 2014;29(1):1–23.
91. Koh JS, Goh SK, Png MA, et al. Femoral cortical stress lesions in long-term bisphosphonate therapy: a herald of impending fracture? J Orthop Trauma 2010; 24(2):75–81.
92. Neviaser AS, Lane JM, Lenart BA, et al. Low-energy femoral shaft fractures associated with alendronate use. J Orthop Trauma 2008;22(5):346–50.
93. Capeci CM, Tejwani NC. Bilateral low-energy simultaneous or sequential femoral fractures in patients on long-term alendronate therapy. J Bone Joint Surg Am 2009;91(11):2556–61.
94. Lin HN, O'Connor JP. Osteoclast depletion with clodronate liposomes delays fracture healing in mice. J Orthop Res 2017;35(8):1699–706.
95. Hao Y, Wang X, Wang L, et al. Zoledronic acid suppresses callus remodeling but enhances callus strength in an osteoporotic rat model of fracture healing. Bone 2015;81:702–11.
96. Larsson S, Fazzalari NL. Anti-osteoporosis therapy and fracture healing. Arch Orthop Trauma Surg 2014;134(2):291–7.
97. Shoji KE, Earp BE, Rozental TD. The effect of bisphosphonates on the clinical and radiographic outcomes of distal radius fractures in women. J Hand Surg Am 2018;43(2):115–22.

98. Gong HS, Song CH, Lee YH, et al. Early initiation of bisphosphonate does not affect healing and outcomes of volar plate fixation of osteoporotic distal radial fractures. J Bone Joint Surg Am 2012;94(19):1729–36.
99. Xue D, Li F, Chen G, et al. Do bisphosphonates affect bone healing? A meta-analysis of randomized controlled trials. J Orthop Surg Res 2014;9:45.
100. Li YT, Cai HF, Zhang ZL. Timing of the initiation of bisphosphonates after surgery for fracture healing: a systematic review and meta-analysis of randomized controlled trials. Osteoporos Int 2015;26(2):431–41.
101. Riek AE, Towler DA. The pharmacological management of osteoporosis. Mo Med 2011;108(2):118–23.
102. Tsai JN, Uihlein AV, Lee H, et al. Teriparatide and denosumab, alone or combined, in women with postmenopausal osteoporosis: the DATA study randomised trial. Lancet 2013;382(9886):50–6.
103. Bushnell BD, Horton JK, McDonald MF, et al. Perioperative medical comorbidities in the orthopaedic patient. J Am Acad Orthop Surg 2008;16(4):216–27.
104. Tashiro T, Pislaru SV, Blustin JM, et al. Perioperative risk of major non-cardiac surgery in patients with severe aortic stenosis: a reappraisal in contemporary practice. Eur Heart J 2014;35(35):2372–81.
105. Brooks-Brunn JA. Predictors of postoperative pulmonary complications following abdominal surgery. Chest 1997;111(3):564–71.
106. Smetana GW, Lawrence VA, Cornell JE, American College of Physicians, et al. Preoperative pulmonary risk stratification for noncardiothoracic surgery: systematic review for the American College of Physicians. Ann Intern Med 2006;144(8):581–95.
107. Archer C, Levy AR, McGregor M. Value of routine preoperative chest x-rays: a meta-analysis. Can J Anaesth 1993;40(11):1022–7.
108. Chung F, Yuan H, Yin L, et al. Elimination of preoperative testing in ambulatory surgery. Anesth Analg 2009;108(2):467–75.
109. Mathew A, Devereaux PJ, O'Hare A, et al. Chronic kidney disease and postoperative mortality: a systematic review and meta-analysis. Kidney Int 2008;73(9):1069–81.
110. Bhattacharyya T, Iorio R, Healy WL. Rate of and risk factors for acute inpatient mortality after orthopaedic surgery. J Bone Joint Surg Am 2002;84-A(4):562–72.
111. Karaeminogullari O, Demirors H, Sahin O, et al. Analysis of outcomes for surgically treated hip fractures in patients undergoing chronic hemodialysis. J Bone Joint Surg Am 2007;89(2):324–31.
112. Corti MC, Guralnik JM, Salive ME, et al. Serum albumin level and physical disability as predictors of mortality in older persons. JAMA 1994;272(13):1036–42.
113. Stone AV, Jinnah A, Wells BJ, et al. Nutritional markers may identify patients with greater risk of re-admission after geriatric hip fractures. Int Orthop 2018;42(2):231–8.
114. Goisser S, Schrader E, Singler K, et al. Malnutrition according to mini nutritional assessment is associated with severe functional impairment in geriatric patients before and up to 6 months after hip fracture. J Am Med Dir Assoc 2015;16(8):661–7.
115. Davis CJ, Sowa D, Keim KS, et al. The use of prealbumin and C-reactive protein for monitoring nutrition support in adult patients receiving enteral nutrition in an urban medical center. JPEN J Parenter Enteral Nutr 2012;36(2):197–204.
116. Kuszajewski ML, Clontz AS. Prealbumin is best for nutritional monitoring. Nursing 2005;35(5):70–1.

117. Smetana GW, Macpherson DS. The case against routine preoperative laboratory testing. Med Clin North Am 2003;87(1):7–40.
118. Guss D, Bhattacharyya T. Perioperative management of the obese orthopaedic patient. J Am Acad Orthop Surg 2006;14(7):425–32.
119. Oberbek J, Synder M. Impact of body mass index (BMI) on early outcomes of total knee arthroplasty. Ortop Traumatol Rehabil 2015;17(2):127–34.
120. Bergin PF, Russell GV. The effects of obesity in orthopaedic care. Instr Course Lect 2015;64:11–24.
121. Jones CA, Cox V, Jhangri GS, et al. Delineating the impact of obesity and its relationship on recovery after total joint arthroplasties. Osteoarthritis Cartilage 2012;20(6):511–8.
122. Poirier P, Alpert MA, Fleisher LA, et al. Cardiovascular evaluation and management of severely obese patients undergoing surgery: a science advisory from the American Heart Association. Circulation 2009;120(1):86–95.
123. Walke LM, Rosenthal RA, Trentalange M, et al. Restructuring care for older adults undergoing surgery: preliminary data from the Co-Management of Older Operative Patients En Route across Treatment Environments (CO-OPERATE) model of care. J Am Geriatr Soc 2014;62(11):2185–90.
124. Huddleston JM, Long KH, Naessens JM, et al. Medical and surgical comanagement after elective hip and knee arthroplasty: a randomized, controlled trial. Ann Intern Med 2004;141(1):28–38.
125. Phy MP, Vanness DJ, Melton LJ 3rd, et al. Effects of a hospitalist model on elderly patients with hip fracture. Arch Intern Med 2005;165(7):796–801.
126. Vazirani S, Lankarani-Fard A, Liang LJ, et al. Perioperative processes and outcomes after implementation of a hospitalist-run preoperative clinic. J Hosp Med 2012;7(9):697–701.
127. Defillo JC, Goncalves Monteiro J, Rubin LE, et al. Impact of a geriatric co-management program for elective joint replacement. Innov Aging 2017; 1(suppl_1):108–9.
128. Auerbach AD, Wachter RM, Cheng HQ, et al. Comanagement of surgical patients between neurosurgeons and hospitalists. Arch Intern Med 2010; 170(22):2004–10.
129. Bini SA, Fithian DC, Paxton LW, et al. Does discharge disposition after primary total joint arthroplasty affect readmission rates? J Arthroplasty 2010;25(1): 114–7.
130. London DA, Vilensky S, O'Rourke C, et al. Discharge disposition after joint replacement and the potential for cost savings: effect of hospital policies and surgeons. J Arthroplasty 2016;31(4):743–8.
131. Ramos NL, Wang EL, Karia RJ, et al. Correlation between physician specific discharge costs, LOS, and 30-day readmission rates: an analysis of 1,831 cases. J Arthroplasty 2014;29(9):1717–22.
132. Chao TF, Liu CJ, Lin YJ, et al. Oral anticoagulation in very elderly patients with atrial fibrillation: a nationwide cohort study. Circulation 2018;138(1):37–47.
133. Desai V, Chan PH, Prentice HA, et al. Is anesthesia technique associated with a higher risk of mortality or complications within 90 days of surgery for geriatric patients with hip fractures? Clin Orthop Relat Res 2018;476(6):1178–88.
134. Olsen F, Kotyra M, Houltz E, et al. Bone cement implantation syndrome in cemented hemiarthroplasty for femoral neck fracture: incidence, risk factors, and effect on outcome. Br J Anaesth 2014;113(5):800–6.
135. Jaidev J. Bone cement implantation syndrome and the surgeon. Br J Anaesth 2016;116(2):303–4.

136. Griffiths R. Bone cement implantation syndrome and the surgeon. Br J Anaesth 2016;116(2):304.
137. de Laat EH, Pickkers P, Schoonhoven L, et al. Guideline implementation results in a decrease of pressure ulcer incidence in critically ill patients. Crit Care Med 2007;35(3):815–20.
138. Dan Berlowitz M, MPH. Prevention of pressure-induced skin and soft tissue injury. 2018. Available at: https://www.uptodate.com/contents/prevention-of-pressure-induced-skin-and-soft-tissue-injury. Accessed April 8, 2018.
139. Sambandam B, Batra S, Gupta R, et al. Blood conservation strategies in orthopedic surgeries: a review. J Clin Orthop Trauma 2013;4(4):164–70.
140. American Academy of Orthopaedic Surgeons. Preventing venous thromboembolic disease in patients undergoing elective hip and knee arthroplasty. Evidence-based guideline and evidence report. Available at: https://www.aaos.org/uploadedFiles/PreProduction/Quality/Guidelines_and_Reviews/VTE_full_guideline_10.31.16.pdf. Accessed April 3, 2018.
141. Biffl WL, Biffl SE. Rehabilitation of the geriatric surgical patient: predicting needs and optimizing outcomes. Surg Clin North Am 2015;95(1):173–90.
142. Chudyk AM, Jutai JW, Petrella RJ, et al. Systematic review of hip fracture rehabilitation practices in the elderly. Arch Phys Med Rehabil 2009;90(2):246–62.
143. Auais MA, Eilayyan O, Mayo NE. Extended exercise rehabilitation after hip fracture improves patients' physical function: a systematic review and meta-analysis. Phys Ther 2012;92(11):1437–51.
144. Latham NK, Harris BA, Bean JF, et al. Effect of a home-based exercise program on functional recovery following rehabilitation after hip fracture: a randomized clinical trial. JAMA 2014;311(7):700–8.
145. Khan F, Ng L, Gonzalez S, et al. Multidisciplinary rehabilitation programmes following joint replacement at the hip and knee in chronic arthropathy. Cochrane Database Syst Rev 2008;(2):CD004957.
146. Gill SD, McBurney H. Does exercise reduce pain and improve physical function before hip or knee replacement surgery? A systematic review and meta-analysis of randomized controlled trials. Arch Phys Med Rehabil 2013;94(1):164–76.

Vascular Surgery and Geriatric Patients

Pegge M. Halandras, MD

KEYWORDS

- Delirium • Frailty • Aortic aneurysm • Carotid artery endarterectomy
- Critical limb ischemia • End stage renal disease

KEY POINTS

- The demand for vascular surgery is expected to be greater than other medical specialties as the population ages.
- Elderly patients scheduled for intervention should be screened for delirium to guide treatment planning.
- Endovascular interventions have expanded treatment options for appropriately selected elderly patients.
- Although a vascular intervention may be feasible, individual medical condition and desired outcomes and expectations should be discussed with elderly patients before surgery.

INTRODUCTION

The world's elderly population continues to grow, and this may be secondary to advancements in health care that promote longevity and healthier existences.[1] Census Bureau data estimate the US population aged 65 years and older is projected to increase from 40.5 million elderly people in 2010 to 89 million people in 2025.[2] The aging of the population can be expected to be accompanied by increased prevalence of chronic disease with multiple comorbidities. In the United States, this change in demographics is expected to result in the greatest projected growth in demand for vascular surgery as compared with other medical specialties. The nature of treatment options for this specialty have continued to advance with improved medical management of risk factors, such as statin therapy, and less invasive endovascular treatment options. These advances in vascular surgery have allowed the specialty to keep pace with the aging population demographic. The true challenge for vascular surgeons rests in the ability to appropriately select patients who will obtain the desired survival benefit for a given surgical intervention.

Disclosure Statement: No disclosure of any relationship with a commercial company that has a direct financial interest in subject matter or materials discussed in the article or with a company making a competing product.
Department of Vascular Surgery and Endovascular Surgery, Loyola University Chicago, Stritch School of Medicine, 2160 South First Avenue, EMS Building 110, Room 3220, Maywood, IL 60153, USA
E-mail address: phalandras@lumc.edu

ANESTHESIA CONSIDERATIONS FOR VASCULAR SURGERY IN ELDERLY PATIENTS

Elderly patients presenting for vascular surgery usually undergo procedures aimed at treating atherosclerotic occlusive disease or aneurysmal disease. Overall, studies have revealed postoperative survival is inversely related to the number of comorbidities.[3] The specific comorbidities are also important; patients undergoing anesthesia for vascular surgery should be carefully assessed for ischemic heart disease, chronic respiratory disease, hypertension, and diabetes mellitus.[4]

Preoperative Assessment

History and physical examination are aimed at identifying signs of left ventricular or congestive cardiac failure and chronic pulmonary disease. Ischemic heart disease may be difficult to identify in this patient population, as a decreased activity level may not provoke ischemia. The role of preoperative provoked myocardial stress testing should be to modify management for reduction of morbidity and mortality. Selected testing should be instituted in patients with severe disease, such as recent myocardial infarction, angina at rest or of increasing severity, or overt cardiac failure. Significant smoking history is also common in vascular surgery patients and can result in respiratory disease. Pulmonary function can be optimized before surgery with the treatment of respiratory infection or symptoms. Moreover, pulmonary function tests are usually reserved for those patients with severe pulmonary compromise and/or those undergoing aortic surgery.[4]

In addition, risk factors for delirium should be assessed in the preoperative period. Delirium is defined as an acute disorder with a transient fluctuating disturbance of consciousness, attention, cognition, and perception. Postoperative delirium has been associated with increased postoperative complications, decreased functional capacity, prolonged length of stay, and increased health care costs.[5] Five independent risk factors have been identified and include baseline dementia, vision impairment, physical restraints, functional impairment, and multiple comorbidities[6] (**Fig. 1**). These risk factors should be recognized in the preoperative period and used to guide clinical decision-making to institute preventative strategies in the postoperative period.

Operative Management

Elderly patients have less physiologic reserve; the aging process results in impaired temperature control, decreased cardiopulmonary reflexes, and a noncompliant vascular tree. Whether patients undergoing vascular surgery receive a general anesthetic, regional anesthetic, or a combination of both, the goals of the anesthetic should be as follows[4,7]:

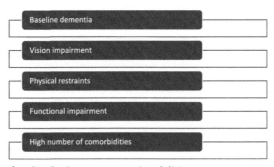

Fig. 1. Risk factors for developing postoperative delirium.

- Avoidance of hypertension, hypotension, and tachycardia
- Maintenance of oxygenation
- Maintenance of blood volume
- Replacement of interstitial and evaporative fluid losses
- Maintenance of body temperature
- Reduction of stress response to surgery
- Optimal oxygen delivery

Postoperative Management

Measures aimed to minimize the risk of postoperative delirium should be used. These measures may include correcting volumes status, treating infections, and providing eye glasses and hearing aids as soon as possible. In addition, a normal sleep-wake cycle should be reestablished.[7]

COMMON VASCULAR SURGERY INTERVENTIONS IN THE ELDERLY

The decision to offer a vascular reconstructive procedure to elderly patients requires thoughtful patient selection and the appropriate procedure that will result in the desired outcome for the patients. This decision-making may be complicated by the fact that interventions can be technically performed with less invasive approaches (endovascular or hybrid approaches) but, because of multiple comorbidities, do not result in acceptable morbidity and mortality rates. Data have shown emergent cases are more prevalent in elderly patients and have a higher morbidity and mortality compared with younger patients.[7,8] These issues complicate the decision whether to offer an elective carotid endarterectomy (CEA) to asymptomatic elderly patients with a high-grade carotid stenosis or older patients with an asymptomatic enlarging abdominal aortic aneurysm.

One tool that may assist surgeons in identifying appropriate patients for surgical intervention is the assessment of frailty. Frailty is a geriatric syndrome of decreased reserve and resistance to stressors resulting from cumulative declines across multiple physiologic systems and causing vulnerability to adverse outcomes. Frailty has been shown to be a risk factor for poor surgical outcomes and can be assessed by the surgeon using a frailty phenotype assessment that takes into account unintentional weight loss, exhaustion, muscle weakness, slowness while walking, and low level of activity. An alternative approach is to assess the deficit accumulation index in which frailty is viewed in terms of the number of health deficits manifested in an individual. Higher frailty scores correlate with higher mortality and morbidity than are acceptable when compared with patients with lower frailty scores for patients receiving the same intervention.[7]

Aortic Aneurysms

Most aortic aneurysms are secondary to age related aortic degenerative pathology. Consequently, the prevalence of abdominal aortic aneurysm (AAA) has increased with the aging of the population. The risk of rupture increases with increasing aneurysm diameter. The Society of Vascular Surgery's guidelines recommend elective repair of an AAA when the diameter is 5.5 cm or greater because the risk of rupture outweighs the operative risk. Two-thirds of AAA ruptures are reported to have occurred in patients 75 years of age or older and are associated with a 30-day mortality risk of 69%.[9] There is considerable debate when considering patient selection based on size criteria and whether reconstruction is performed via an endovascular or open approach.

The Society for Vascular Surgery's Vascular Quality Initiative (VQI) database was used to compare mortality rates in patients 80 years of age and older undergoing either an endovascular AAA repair (EVAR) or open AAA repair (OAR) to younger patients from 2002 to 2012. Perioperative mortality was higher in both the OAR and EVAR octogenarian group as compared with the younger patients. The 1-year mortality rate was also higher for the elderly independent of the type of repair when compared with the younger group (**Table 1**). The higher perioperative and 1-year mortality rates in the octogenarian group led the investigators to suggest that the size criteria used to select patients for an OAR be greater than 5.5 cm because of the greater operative risk in this older group. Multivariate analysis also confirmed the strongest predictors associated with perioperative and 1-year mortality rates regardless of the type of AAA repair were age greater than 79 years, emergent/urgent repair, and need for postoperative vasopressor agents.[10] This finding highlights the importance of careful consideration before proceeding with repair of a ruptured aneurysm in octogenarians.

The less invasive nature of EVAR seems to offer a tempting solution for elective repair of an AAA in octogenarians. To validate this approach, a meta-analysis and systematic review of short-term and midterm outcomes in octogenarians versus younger patients undergoing EVAR for AAA treatment was completed. Nine observational studies were included. The older group had a higher incidence of comorbidities and a higher American Society of Anesthesiologist score. The technical success rate was similar between the two groups. The investigators included the differences in the anatomy of the aneurysm and procedural data for both groups. The older patients had a larger aneurysm diameter, but the neck length and diameter were similar for the two groups. The operative time, blood loss, and hospital length of stay were statistically higher in the elderly group. Although the 30-day mortality rate for the two groups was not statistically different, it was lower for the octogenarians (1.68% vs 3.73%, respectively). In contrast, the 1-year mortality rate was significantly higher for the elderly (9.16% vs 4.47%, respectively).[11] This review confirms a poorer long-term outcome for older patients undergoing EVAR. It also suggests EVAR may offer a valid treatment option for appropriately selected elderly patients.

Carotid Artery Stenosis

The management of carotid occlusive disease in the elderly has not been studied. The North American Symptomatic Carotid Endarterectomy Trial (NASCET) and the Asymptomatic Carotid Atherosclerosis Study (ACAS) both excluded patients older than 80 years because of presumed elevated perioperative risk and limited life expectancy. These studies established the foundation for carotid stenosis treatment algorithms in younger patients. Therefore, in the past, CEA was not routinely recommended to older patients because it was thought that there was no benefit because of an assumed limited life expectancy. One subsequent retrospective study evaluated 334 patients 80 years of age or older compared with 1627 younger patients undergoing CEA between 1993 and 2004. There was no difference in stroke risk between the two groups, but there was an increased mortality rate in the older group. In addition, the combined risk for stroke/death was greater in the symptomatic older patients. This study confirmed CEA was safe and effective in octogenarians, as perioperative outcomes were within standards established in national guidelines and also confer a benefit for reduced risk for stroke.[12]

Schneider and colleagues[13] reported outcomes for CEA in elderly patients using the Society for Vascular Surgery's VQI database from 2003 to 2015. There were 7390 elderly patients (>80 years old) who underwent a CEA. This group was compared

Table 1
Outcomes for octogenarians versus nonoctogenarians undergoing OAR and EVAR

Outcome	OAR (n = 5765)			EVAR (n = 16,109)			Overall (N = 21,874)		
	Nonoctogenarian (n = 5000; 87%)	Octogenarian (n = 765; 13%)	P Value	Nonoctogenarian (n = 12,035; 13%)	Octogenarian (n = 4074; 25%)	P Value	Nonoctogenarian (n = 17,035; 78%)	Octogenarian (n = 4839; 22%)	P Value
Perioperative (30 d) mortality	7.1	20.1	<.01	1.6	3.8	<.01	3.2	6.4	<.01
Elective repair	2.8	6.7	<.01	0.6	1.6	<.01	1.2	2.2	<.01
Emergent repair	19.4	40.8	<.01	8.2	17.4	<.01	13.2	25.5	<.01
1-y All-cause mortality	9.7	26.0	<.01	4.3	8.9	<.01	5.9	11.6	<.01
Elective repair	5.0	11.9	<.01	2.9	6.2	<.01	3.4	6.9	<.01
Emergent repair	23.0	47.8	<.01	13.3	25.5	<.01	17.7	33.2	<.01

Data are shown in percentages.
Bold values indicate statistical significance ($P < .05$).
From Hicks CW, Obeid T, Arhuidese I, et al. Abdominal aortic aneurysm repair in octogenarians is associated with higher mortality compared with nonoctogenarians. J Vasc Surg 2016;64:960; with permission.

with 35,303 younger patients. The neurologic complication and perioperative myocardial infarction rates were higher in the elderly who were also more likely to be discharged to either long-term care or a rehabilitation facility. In addition, Kaplan-Meier analysis estimated survival at 30 days and 1 year was lower for the group older than 79 years. Therefore, the investigators recommended considering CEA in intellectually intact independent older patients with a high-grade stenosis who seem to have a significant life expectancy.

In contrast to other vascular disease processes, endovascular stenting for carotid stenosis in older patients is not supported by current data. This recommendation of avoiding carotid stenting in older patients is based on a 12.1% procedural stroke rate observed in the initial phase of Carotid Revascularization Endarterectomy versus Stenting Trial (CREST). The investigators thought this finding was related to the increased aortic atherosclerotic plaque burden and difficult arch anatomy that is, common in the elderly. This early finding resulted in octogenarians being excluded from further enrollment in the trial.[14]

Lower Extremity Ischemia

Peripheral arterial disease occurs in up to 15% to 20% in the elderly population.[15] This disease entity has several stages ranging from lifestyle-limiting claudication to critical limb ischemia (CLI) defined as ischemic rest pain and/or nonhealing wounds.

A retrospective review of the Healthcare Cost and Utilization Project Nationwide Inpatient Sample was used to identify patients with a diagnosis of lifestyle-limiting claudication due to infrainguinal disease that were treated by either open or endovascular revascularization. The time period spanned from 2003 to 2012; patients were grouped according to age, including 60 to 80 years of age or older than 80 years. In contrast to the young cohort, the proportion of endovascular interventions in the octogenarian group transitioned during the study period to 60% with the remaining 40% receiving an open procedure (**Fig. 2**). Overall, exacerbation of congestive heart failure,

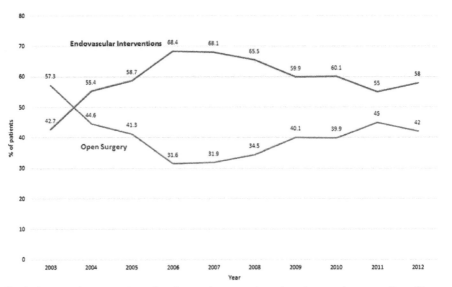

Fig. 2. Increase in proportion of endovascular procedures in octogenarians over time. (*From* Erben Y, Mena-Hurtado CI, Miller SM, et al. Increased mortality in octogenarians treated for lifestyle limiting claudication. Catheter Cardiovasc Interv 2018;91:1335; with permission.)

acute kidney injury, mortality rate, and proportion of patients discharged to a skilled nursing facility was higher in octogenarians compared with the younger cohort independent of the approach used for revascularization. Lifestyle-limiting claudication is recognized as having a low risk for adverse limb outcomes, and mortality rates in this study were less than 1% for both groups. Despite this overall low rate for the entire study population, the mortality rate was higher in the octogenarians. Therefore, management must also include conservative therapy (supervised exercise programs and maximal medical management) in addition to open or endovascular revascularization techniques.[16]

In contrast to this low risk of adverse events with interventions for claudication, treatment of CLI is focused on revascularization to relieve ischemic rest pain and prevent limb loss. A prospective study evaluated the difference in outcomes between 2 age groups, 70 to 79 years old and greater than 80 years old, with critical limb ischemia. There were 3 study groups, including nonoperative and open or endovascular revascularization. Nonoperative therapy consisted of pharmacologic treatment of pain, intensive wound care, and minor amputations. The primary end point measured was the quality of life (QoL), and the secondary end points were mortality rate and limb salvage. The overall 6-month limb salvage rate was 79%, and 6-month mortality rate was significantly lower in the patients receiving an open procedure (7%) as compared with the endovascular group (32%) and conservative group (26%). Additionally, the amputation-free survival was significantly higher in the surgically treated group. The younger cohort group experienced the most benefit from surgical revascularization with lower mortality rates, lower adverse events, and improved QoL at the 1-week, 6-week, and 6-month evaluations. The older cohort had no difference in mortality and limb salvage rates between the 3 treatment arms, but physical health improved at 6 weeks postoperatively in those treated by either an open or endovascular intervention. This improvement was not seen until 6 months after initiation of medical treatment in the nonoperative group. These results suggest that surgical revascularization is superior to other treatments in carefully selected elderly patients with CLI.[15]

Hemodialysis Access

The elderly represent the fastest growing segment of the incident hemodialysis population.[17] Creation of hemodialysis access in the elderly represents a complicated decision-making process. A physician must consider multiple issues, including placement of the most appropriate hemodialysis access type, predicting patients' life expectancy, the likelihood of progressing to needing dialysis before death, and patient preference. This decision-making process should involve a multidisciplinary approach including the patients and their families, the nephrologist, and the surgeon.

Progression to end-stage renal disease (ESRD) is not a standardized event, and research has been focused on an attempt to identify those elderly patients who will need hemodialysis before death. A Veterans Affairs' (VA) study that included 2,583,911 veterans with at least one serum creatinine investigated the association between estimated glomerular filtration rate (eGFR) and survival rates in different age groups. In the 18- to 44-year-old group, the risk of ESRD exceeded the risk of death if the eGFR was less than 45 mL/min/1.73 m². For those in the 65- to 84-year-old group, the risk of ESRD exceeded the risk of death if eGFR was lower than or equal to 15 mL/min/1.73 m² In contrast, the risk of death persistently exceeded the risk of ESRD in those 85 years of age or older.[18] This highlights the importance of the limited life expectancy in octogenarians with chronic renal disease.

Once the decision has been made that hemodialysis will benefit older patients, the optimal access must be determined. Patients may be candidates for an

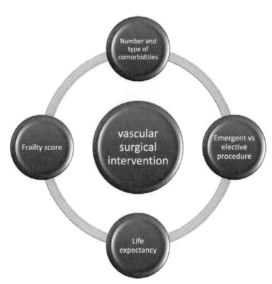

Fig. 3. Factors to consider before offering a vascular procedure in elderly patients.

arteriovenous fistula (AVF), an arteriovenous graft (AVG), or a central venous catheter. Elderly patients with minimal comorbidities with an expected hemodialysis start date more than 6 months after creation of the access may be an excellent candidate for AVF placement because there will be adequate time for the fistula to mature. If elderly patients have a more limited life expectancy of 1 to 2 years and multiple comorbidities, an AVG may be a better choice. This access may be used sooner and avoid central venous catheter placement.[19] Finally, a central venous catheter, which is typically the least desired option, may be a better choice for patients with a limited life expectancy, multiple comorbidities, and an acute need for hemodialysis.

SUMMARY

The aging of the population is creating profound changes in the specialty of vascular surgery. Previous procedures that were prohibitive in elderly patients with multiple comorbidities have been replaced by less invasive endovascular or hybrid procedures. These new advances in surgery and the trend for increased longevity have made the art of practicing vascular surgery much more complex. Although a vascular procedure may be technically feasible, a patient's and the desired outcome should be thoroughly assessed in the preoperative period. Factors to consider before surgery include a patient's frailty score, the number and type of comorbidities, emergent or elective nature of procedure, and the patient's life expectancy (**Fig. 3**). Identification of goals of therapy and discussion of possible outcomes, such as discharge to other than home after intervention, should be frankly discussed. In conclusion, this shared decision-making should assist patients, the patient's support system, and the surgeon in making a treatment plan with the highest chance of achieving the desired outcome.

REFERENCES

1. Kassahun WT, Staab H, Gockel I, et al. Factors associated with morbidity and in-hospital mortality after surgery beyond the age of 90:, comparison with outcome

results of younger patients matched for treatment. Am J Surg 2017. https://doi. org/10.1016/j.amjsurg.2017.11.032.

2. Dall TM, Gallo PD, Chakrabarti R, et al. An aging population and growing disease burden will require a large and specialized health care workforce by 2025. Health Aff 2013;32(11):2013–20.

3. Hosking MP, Warner MA, Lobdell CM, et al. Outcomes of surgery in patients 90 years of age and older. JAMA 1989;261(13):1909–15.

4. Wilkins CJ. Anaesthesia and vascular surgery in the elderly. Curr Anaesth Crit Care 1997;8:113–9.

5. Raats JW, Steunenberg SL, de Lange DC, et al. Risk factors of post-operative delirium after elective vascular surgery in the elderly: a systematic review. Int J Surg 2016;35:1–6.

6. Inouye SK, Zhang Y, Jones RN, et al. Risk factors for delirium at discharge: development and validation of a predictive model. Arch Intern Med 2007;167(13): 1406–13.

7. Johanning JM, Matthew Longo G, Melin AA. Preoperative optimization of the elderly patient prior to vascular surgery. In: Chaer R, editor. Vascular Disease in Older Adults. Cham (Switzerland): Springer; 2017. p. 35–43.

8. Linn BS, Linn MW, Wallen N. Evaluation of results of surgical procedures in the elderly. Ann Surg 1982;195:90–6.

9. Howard DP, Banerjee A, Fairhead JF, et al, Oxford Vascular Study. Age-specific incidence, risk factors and outcome of acute abdominal aortic aneurysms in a defined population. Br J Surg 2015;102(8):907–15.

10. Hicks CW, Obeid T, Arhuidese I, et al. Abdominal aortic aneurysm repair in octogenarians is associated with higher mortality compared with nonoctogenarians. J Vasc Surg 2016;64:956–65.

11. Han Y, Zhang S, Zhang J, et al. Outcome of endovascular abdominal aortic aneurysm repair in octogenarians: meta-analysis and systemic review. Eur J Vasc Endovasc Surg 2017;54:454–63.

12. Miller MT, Comerota AJ, Tzilinis A, et al. Carotid endarterectomy in octogenarians: does increased age indicate "high risk"? J Vasc Surg 2005;41:231–7.

13. Schneider JR, Jackson CR, Helenowski IB, et al. A comparison of results of carotid endarterectomy in octogenarians and nonagenarians to younger patients from the mid-America vascular study group and the society for vascular surgery vascular quality initiative. J Vasc Surg 2017;65:1643–52.

14. Faggioli G, Ferri M, Rapezzi C, et al. Atherosclerotic aortic lesions increase the risk of cerebral embolism during carotid stenting in patients with complex aortic arch anatomy. J Vasc Surg 2009;49:80–5.

15. Steunenberg SL, de Vries J, Raats JW, et al. Quality of life and mortality after endovascular, surgical or conservative treatment of elderly patients suffering from critical limb ischemia. Ann Vasc Surg 2018;51:95–105.

16. Erben Y, Mena-Hurtado CI, Miller SM, et al. Increased mortality in octogenarians treated for lifestyle limiting claudication. Catheter Cardiovasc Interv 2018;91: 1331–8.

17. Berger JR, Jaikaransingh V, Hedayati SS. End-stage kidney disease in the elderly: approach to dialysis initiation, choosing modality and predicting outcomes. Adv Chronic Kidney Dis 2016;23:36–43.

18. O'Hare AM, Choi AI, Bertenthal D, et al. Age affects outcomes in chronic kidney disease. J Am Soc Nephrol 2007;18:2758–65.

19. Allon M, Lok CE. Dialysis fistula or graft: the role for randomized clinical trials. Clin J Am Soc Nephrol 2010;5(12):2348–54.

Elder Abuse

Astrid Botty Van Den Bruele, MD, Moustapha Dimachk, MD,
Marie Crandall, MD, MPH*

KEYWORDS

- Elder abuse • Family violence • Domestic violence • Financial abuse
- Emotional abuse

KEY POINTS

- Elder abuse is a global problem warranting a global solution; elder abuse is predicted to increase because many countries are experiencing rapidly aging populations.
- The lowest prevalence rates of elder abuse are in the United States and Canada. and the highest prevalence rates of elder abuse are in Asia and Nigeria; however, the prevalence rate of elder abuse is likely to be a gross underestimation because many cases of elder abuse go unreported.
- Impairment/dementia, poor mental health, low income/socioeconomic strata, financial dependence, gender, age, and race/ethnicity are some of the most commonly cited risk factors for elder abuse.
- Family, friends, and others in a position of trust and authority have been recognized to be potential perpetrators of abuse.
- Creation and development of adequate screening protocols help in identifying individuals at risk for abuse, but are imperfect and subject to interpretation.

INTRODUCTION

Elder abuse is increasingly being recognized as a global public health concern and social problem.[1] The most recent estimates suggest that approximately 4.3 million older individuals experience one or more forms of elder abuse annually.[1,2] Elder abuse is generally defined as the maltreatment of individuals over the age of 60. However, a major obstacle to improving the understanding of elder abuse has been due to the lack of a unanimous definition. Fortunately, consensus is now emerging regarding the general definition of elder abuse as well as the major types of mistreatment.[3] Types of abuse include emotional, sexual, physical, and financial.[1]

The World Health Organization (WHO) recognizes elder abuse as a single, or repeated, act or acts or even a lack of appropriate action/intervention, occurring within

Disclosure Statement: The authors have nothing to disclose.
Department of Surgery, University of Florida College of Medicine Jacksonville, 655 West 8th Street, Jacksonville, FL 32209, USA
* Corresponding author.
E-mail address: marie.crandall@jax.ufl.edu

any relationship where there is an expectation of trust, which causes harm or distress to an older person.[4] The WHO estimates that 15.7% of people 60 years and older are subjected to abuse.[4] However, the prevalence rate is likely to be an underestimation because many cases of elder abuse go unreported. Evidence suggests that only a fraction of cases actually get referred to the appropriate social services agencies.[5] A meta-analysis by Ho and colleagues[6] revealed that third parties or caregivers were more likely to report abuse than the abused individual himself or herself. The pooled prevalence of elder abuse was estimated to be 10.0% and 34.3% in population-based studies and third party–reported or caregiver-reported studies, respectively.[6]

Elder abuse is associated with significant morbidity and premature mortality. Although some markers of elder abuse are more apparent than others, older victims often experience numerous adverse health effects that may not be immediately evident and persist long after the abuse has stopped.[7] The long-term effects of elder abuse include new or exacerbated health problems, premature institutionalization, and a hastened death.[8–11] General risk factors associated with physical and sexual abuse include female gender, social isolation, multiple chronic comorbidities, and having a caregiver who is experiencing stress, who has substance abuse issues, or who displays poor coping skills.[12–22] The perpetrators are usually family members, friends, and others they trust and rely on. The close relationship between perpetrator and victim is exploited and manipulated due to its vulnerability and dependence. With the increase in the aging population globally, there is an increase in the number of individuals who may require additional care and support as a result of their circumstances. Although some caretakers welcome the opportunity to care for their aging loved ones, others may feel as if this places an additional burden on families and society as a whole.

Elder abuse is a global phenomenon and, without proper recognition and intervention, is only anticipated to worsen with the aging population. As many countries are experiencing rapidly aging populations, the number of people affected is predicted to increase. By 2030, more than 20% of US residents are projected to be aged 65 and over.[8] Unfortunately, this creates an even larger and more vulnerable population for exploitation.

MATERIALS AND METHODS

A literature review search was performed. Three databases were searched: PubMed, MEDLINE, and Cochrane. Three meSH terms were used, "elder abuse," "elder maltreatment," and "perpetrator characteristics." To ensure a more global representation, articles with data based on population from different geographic areas were also selected.

The resultant data were then used to identify risk factors for abuse, types of abuse, differences in prevalence among geographic regions, gender, and socioeconomic status as well as current screening tools using prevention. A flowchart describing the process of study selection is shown in **Fig. 1**.

RESULTS

Elder abuse does not have a consensus definition within the literature, and the lack of unanimity likely contributes to different risk estimations. A large meta-analysis conducted by Ho and colleagues[6] included 34 studies with a total of just over 44.5 million participants globally, more than 3 times that reported in previous population-based studies. Subgroup analyses found emotional abuse to be the most common, with

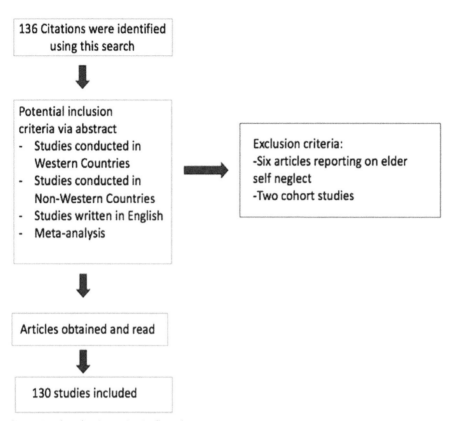

Fig. 1. Study selection criteria flowchart.

estimated prevalence of 47.5%, followed by financial and physical abuse with prevalence rates of 34% and 19.1%, respectively.[6] Sexual abuse was the least often reported with a prevalence rate of just 3%.[6] However, similar to sexual abuse in other age groups and communities, this seemingly lower incidence may reflect failure to screen or lack of disclosure by victims.

RISK FACTORS

Certain patient-level risk factors exist that are associated with a higher likelihood of elder abuse. Functional dependence, disability, cognitive impairment, low socioeconomic status, financial dependence, gender, age, and race/ethnicity are some of the most commonly cited risk factors seen within the literature (**Fig. 2**).

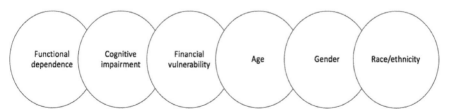

Fig. 2. Risk factors for abuse.

Disability, both cognitive and physical, is known to be associated with increased risk of abuse.[1] In a review of the literature, Pillemer and colleagues[3] posited that disability is one of the strongest risk factors for abuse. As the risk of dementia and cognitive impairment increases with age, an elderly individual with dementia may not be capable of living independently. Increased dependence may lead to a higher likelihood of being placed into assisted living facilities or nursing homes, and rates of abuse may be higher for older people living in institutions versus the community.[4] The WHO recently conducted a survey of nursing-home staff in the United States. The study reported that 36% of staff admitted to witnessing at least one incident of physical abuse of an elderly patient in the previous year; 10% committed at least one act of physical abuse, and 40% admitted to psychologically abusing patients.[4]

Female gender appears to be at least a potential risk factor for abuse,[3] as Ho and colleagues[6] indicated that women were more likely than men to be abused (17.0% for women vs 10.9% for men). There is speculation that women are more likely to be abused because they have a longer lifespan that is in turn associated with loss of independence in activities of daily living as well as increasing cognitive impairment.[6] In some cultures, there is also thought that women might also be more "socially trained" to endure abuse. A large global literature review performed by Pillemer and colleagues[3] delved into this topic further. The article focused on international studies that indicated that women are more likely than men to experience elder abuse, specifically, emotionally and financially. However, demonstrating that there may be cultural differences in incidence and/or reporting, a recent study conducted in Korea found that men were more likely to experience emotional and financial abuse.[23] These cultural differences have also been found in other areas of research. For example, African Americans may be at increased risk of financial abuse and psychological abuse,[24,25] whereas Hispanic older adults have shown lower risk of emotional abuse, financial abuse, and neglect.[24,26,27] These discrepancies may be regional or cultural, and additional research is warranted to adequately assess the ethnic and cultural ideologies that could influence abuse perceptions and outcomes.

TYPES OF ABUSE

Detecting elder abuse accurately is inherently difficult, because it is often perpetrated against vulnerable individuals by those whom they rely on the most. The Conflict Tactics Scale (CTS) is the most frequently used measurement of abuse within relationships.[28] The modified CTS was created in order to report validity and acceptability of family caregiver self-reports and compare them with interviewer measures of abuse. It found that disabled elders and family caregivers agreed 71% of the time about whether caregivers behaved in an abusive manner.[29]

Although abuse can occur in multiple forms, some of the more recognized examples of abuse include emotional, psychological, physical, financial, and sexual. Of these, the most common subtype is emotional (annual prevalence globally estimated to be 0.7–27.3),[9] followed by financial abuse (annual global prevalence 1.0%–13.1%), physical abuse (0.2%–14.6%), and finally, sexual abuse (0.4%–3.3%), as shown in **Table 1**.

Emotional Abuse

Emotional abuse is inflicting mental stress by actions and threats.[11,30–35] Emotional abuse takes multiple forms and carries with it feelings of unworthiness, embarrassment, and shame, which can further propagate social isolation, a well-known risk factor for abuse. Threatening to place an elder in a nursing home, verbal abuse, and tactics of humiliation are just some examples of emotional abuse.[9,11] As one can

Table 1 Types of abuse	
Types of Abuse	Examples
Financial	Deprivation of food, shelter, and access to health care, stealing
Emotional	Mental stress, bullying, intimidation
Physical	Pain, injury
Sexual	Sexual assault and molestation

imagine, if an elderly individual is experiencing incontinence, ridiculing him/her for the incontinence, especially in a public forum, can be very damaging to their psyche.

Financial Abuse

One of the most frightening scenarios for any person is the possibility of financial ruin and financial dependence is a known contributing factor for abuse.[3] Elders may feel trapped within their environment and, without financial freedom, unable to escape. Financial exploitation/abuse has been described as the fastest growing form of elder abuse.[24] Although not systematically assessed, losing assets accumulated over a lifetime, often through hard work and sacrifice, can be absolutely devastating.[36] In a recent large-scale meta-analysis, Burnes and colleagues[37] estimated that each year, 5.4% (approximately 1 of every 18) of cognitively intact older adults in the United States are victims of financial fraud. The US News and World Report recently reported that seniors lose nearly $36.5 billion to financial abuse annually. A previous widely cited estimate from MetLife put the figure at less than one-tenth of that: still a high loss, at $2.9 billion, but many experts say that is most certainly a gross underestimate, given how very few financial exploitation cases are publicized.[38] Because prevention and recognition are of paramount importance in financial abuse cases, screening tools are currently in development to help identify those susceptible to this abuse. A recent review by Phelan and colleagues[39,40] assessed whether the Older Adult Financial Exploitation Measure could be used as a national safeguarding tool for individuals at risk for financial exploitation. They concluded that this measure lead to a higher suspicion of financial abuse and assisted in identifying instances of possible financial exploitation in a single individual.[41]

Physical Abuse

Perhaps the most egregious type of abuse, physical abuse, is defined as the intentional act resulting in pain, injury, or coercion[11] of an elder individual. Examples include physically hitting, restraining, or injuring said individual.[9] Elder abuse can lead to serious physical injuries and long-term psychological consequences.[4] Worsened functional status, progressive dependency, stress, and further psychological decline are just some of the consequences known to occur.[42] Other medical implications of abuse include increased health care system utilization,[42] and, perhaps most importantly, elder physical abuse is an independent predictor for mortality.[42] It has been estimated that elders who experienced abuse, even modest abuse, had a 300% higher risk of death when compared with those who had not been abused.[43] Demographic characteristics, such as being unmarried, having low educational attainment and low income, have been repeatedly documented in the literature to be associated with elder abuse.[44,45] In the United States, Kentucky and New Jersey rank highest in elder abuse, gross neglect, and exploitation complaints.[46] Canada reported the lowest prevalence rate of 0.5%, whereas Nigeria has the highest measured prevalence rate of 14.6%.[3]

Sexual Abuse

No form of elder abuse is as misrepresented and underreported as that of sexual abuse, with a prevalence rate of just 0.04% to 0.08%.[3,28,47–49] Sexual abuse includes nonconsensual or sexual acts, such as rape, molestation, or exploitative behavior.[9,11] Sexual abuse has both physical and nonphysical components, which may or may not be completely transparent to the observer. Physical signs of sexual abuse include sustaining pelvic injuries, contracting a sexually transmitted disease, bruising within the inner thighs, and genital and/or anal bleeding. Some nonphysical characteristics of sexual abuse include new onset panic attacks, posttraumatic stress disorder, and social or emotional isolation. A recent research investigation on the sexual victimization of older adults living in nursing homes has reported that victims are primarily women and the alleged perpetrators are likely men.[49] Most of the victims seen in that study were more likely to suffer from cognitive deficits or marked physical disability,[50] which likely contributes to the limited reporting of these heinous acts. Data obtained from Acierno and colleagues[1] showed that history of previous traumatic events and low social support to be predictive of sexual abuse (odds ratio 13.98 and 5.68, respectively). Future studies should investigate sexual abuse of vulnerable adults in both facility and community settings.

PERPETRATOR CHARACTERISTICS

The relationship between perpetrators of elder abuse and the abuse victim is quite complex. Elder abuse can take place in any setting and can be inflicted by any person holding a position of trust.[28] Family members, friends, and caretakers have been recognized as potential perpetrators of abuse. Unfortunately, the empirical literature provides little information about perpetrators and their motivations for the abuse.[26]

Adult children who are abusive may be dependent on their parents financially.[29] Not surprisingly, factors underlying dependency in adulthood include substance abuse, a history of mental or emotional illness, and unemployment, which are also risk factors for abuse perpetration.[23,24,36]

As mentioned previously, elder abuse continues to be a global problem warranting a global solution. In 2009, the project on abuse of elderly in Europe (ABUEL) was conducted in 7 European cities to further address this growing crisis and its contributing variables. A 2014 study by Fraga and colleagues[51] analyzed this data further to address the socioeconomic and educational characteristics of the participants. They concluded that there is both a societal and a community level dimension that contributes to individual variability in explaining differences among nations in elder abuse, further highlighting how underlying socioeconomic inequalities lead to such behavior.

SCREENING

With increasing awareness of elder abuse, there has been a push toward the creation and development of adequate screening protocols. The current recommendation from the American Medical Association is that all geriatric patients receive elder abuse screening.[52–55] Unfortunately, there is currently no gold standard for elder abuse screening tools, although there are several that have been validated and are currently in use. The Elder Abuse Suspicion Index (EASI) was designed to increase a provider's suspicion regarding elder abuse. If the provider feels that the individual is experiencing abuse based on the EASI, that provider may propose a referral for further evaluation by social services, adult protective services, or equivalent agencies. The EASI has been shown to have content validity in 7 diverse countries[4] and is currently in use today.

A second tool, the Hwalek-Sengstock Elder Abuse Screening Test, was developed to screen for abuse and may be administered by self-report or interview by a health care professional and has been found to be particularly useful in the emergency or outpatient setting.[37] The Vulnerability to Abuse Screening Scale is used to identity women at risk for elder abuse. It is a self-reported questionnaire of dependency, dejection, coercion, and vulnerability.[39,56] A positive screen for elder abuse does not ubiquitously mean abuse is occurring, but it does indicate that further information should be gathered.

PREVENTION

The global population of people aged 60 years and older will more than double, from 900 million in 2015 to about 2 billion in 2050.[4] Elder abuse is predicted to concomitantly increase.[4] Investing in elderly health and well-being initiatives to keep elderly individuals as independent as long as possible can assist in combating this egregious abuse of the geriatric population. Studies from the United States and Europe have shown that a shared living environment is a major risk factor for aggregated elder abuse and, more specifically, physical and financial abuse.[13,57,58] If an elderly individual can stay independent, the incidence of elder abuse may start to decline. Social support programs promoting healthy living, exercise, and dieting have promising results in regard to physical and mental health. These interventions can lead to decrease in comorbidities, polypharmacy, and depression. In addition, community outreach programs promoting group activities can also assist in decreasing elder abuse, as studies conducted in the United States, Canada, Europe, and Israel have found that higher levels of social support and greater embeddedness in a social network lower the risk of elder abuse.

DISCUSSION

Elder abuse takes a tremendous toll on individuals, families, and communities globally. Its multifactorial cause, vague definition, and lack of precise epidemiology create additional obstacles, which need to be overcome. Just like any challenge, it is difficult to develop a solution if the problem itself cannot be fully identified. The authors propose offering a standardized definition as to what constitutes elder abuse. Elder abuse can be defined as any abuse or exploitation of older individuals aged 65 and over. This abuse would include financial, physical, emotional, or any other situation that leaves the individual susceptible to harm or exploitation based on age.

Second, social support programs for elderly individuals should be expanded. These programs could assist in educating elders that they are in a potentially harmful situation and enlighten them regarding safe alternatives. However, limitations here are vast because the elderly individual (or a third-party individual) must be cognizant of what is happening to him or her. This almost certainly precludes individuals with dementia or any other medical comorbidity in which the individual loses the situational awareness due to cognitive deficits. In this case, it would be up to a third-party individual to report the abuse.

One of the key challenges in this field is developing methods for detection in cognitively impaired older adults. For these impaired populations, researchers must use more indirect methods, such as caregiver or potential perpetrator surveys, health care provider screening tools, reports from social service providers, or other individuals who come into frequent contact with older adults, as well as forensic analysis of bruising patterns.[59,60] With increased education, screening tools, community involvement, and changing social policies, elder abuse can go from being a shameful and dreaded daily reality to becoming distant memory: a problem fixed by mutual understanding, concern, and respect for all individuals across the globe.

REFERENCES

1. Acierno R, Hernandez-Tejada M, Muzzy W, et al. National elder mistreatment study. U. S. Department of Justice; 2009. Available at: https://www.ncjrs.gov/pdffiles1/nij/grants/226456.pdf.
2. Kaplan DB, Pillemer K. Fulfilling the promise of the Elder Justice Act: priority goals for the white house conference on aging. Public Policy Aging Rep 2015;25:63–6.
3. Pillemer K, Burnes D, Riffin C, et al. Elder abuse: global situation, risk factors, and prevention strategies. Gerontologist 2016;56(S2):S194–205.
4. World Health Organization. Available at: http://www.who.int/ageing/projects/elder_abuse/en/. Accessed May 11, 2018.
5. Baker P, Francis D, Hairi NN, et al. Interventions for preventing abuse in the elderly. Cochrane Database Syst Rev 2016;(8):CD010321.
6. Ho CSH, Wong SY, Chiu MM, et al. Global prevalence of elder abuse: a meta-analysis and meta-regression. East Asian Arch Psychiatry 2017;27:43–55.
7. Roberto K. The complexities of elder abuse. Am Psychol 2016;71(4):302–11.
8. Dong X, Simon MA. Elder abuse as a risk factor for hospitalization in older persons. JAMA Intern Med 2013;173:911–7.
9. Luo Y, Waite LJ. Mistreatment and psychological well-being among older adults: exploring the role of psychosocial resources and deficits. J Gerontol B Psychol Sci Soc Sci 2011;66B:217–29.
10. Rovi S, Chen PH, Vega M, et al. Mapping the elder mistreatment iceberg: U.S. hospitalizations with elder abuse and neglect diagnoses. J Elder Abuse Negl 2009;21:346–59.
11. Baker MW, LaCroix AZ, Wu C, et al. Mortality risk associated with physical and verbal abuse in women aged 50 to 79. J Am Geriatr Soc 2009;57:1799–809.
12. Friedman LS, Avila S, Tanouye K, et al. A case-control study of severe physical abuse of the elderly. J Am Geriatr Soc 2011;59:417–22.
13. Acierno R, Hernandez MA, Amstadter AB, et al. Prevalence and correlates of emotional, physical, sexual, and financial abuse and potential neglect in the United States: the national elder mistreatment study. Am J Public Health 2010;100:292–7.
14. Lachs MS, Pillemer K. Elder abuse. Lancet 2004;364:1263–72.
15. Dong X, Simon MA, Gorbien M, et al. Loneliness in older Chinese adults: a risk factor for elder mistreatment. J Am Geriatr Soc 2007;55:1831–5.
16. Cooper C, Selwood A, Blanchard M, et al. The determinants of family cargivers' abusive behaviour to people with dementia: results of the CARD study. J Affect Disord 2010;121:136–42.
17. Livingston G, Barber J, Rapaport P, et al. Clinical effectiveness of a manual based coping strategy programme (START, STrAtegies for RelaTives) in promoting the mental health of carers of family members with dementia: pragmatic randomised controlled trial. BMJ 2013;347:f6276.
18. Anetzberger G, Korbin J, Austin C. Alcoholism and elder abuse. J Interpers Violence 1994;9:184–93.

19. Reay AM, Browne KD. Risk factor characteristics in carers who physically abuse or neglect their elderly dependents. Aging Ment Health 2001;5:56–62.

20. Pillemer K, Suitor JJ. Violence and violent feelings: what causes them among family givers? J Gerontol 1992;47:S165–72.

21. Dong XQ, Simon MA, Beck TT, et al. Elder abuse and mortality: the role of psychological and social wellbeing. Gerontology 2011;57:549–58.

22. Cisler JM, Amstadter AB, Begle AM, et al. Elder mistreatment and physical health among older adults: the South Carolina Elder Mistreatment Study. J Trauma Stress 2010;23:461–7.

23. Burnett J, Jackson SL, Sinha AK, et al. Five-year all-cause mortality rates across five categories of substantiated elder abuse occurring in the community. J Elder Abuse Negl 2016;28(2):59–75.

24. Cooper C, Manela M, Katona C, et al. Screening for elder abuse in dementia in the LASER-AD study; prevalence, correlated and validation of instruments. Int J Geriatr Psychiatry 2008;23:283–8.

25. Beach SR, Schulz R, Williamson GM, et al. Risk factors for potetionally harmful information caregiver behavior. J Am Geriatr Soc 2005;53(2):255–61.

26. Oh J, Kim HS, Martins D, et al. A study of elder abuse in Korea. Int J Nurs Stud 2006;43:203–14. https://doi.org/10.1016/j.ijnurstu.2005.03.005.

27. Hafemeiser T. Elder mistreatment: abuse, neglect, and exploitation in an aging America, vol. 13. NIH; 2003.

28. Burnes D, Pillemer K, Caccamise PL, et al. Prevalence of and risk factors for elder abuse and neglect in the community: a population-based study. J Am Geriatr Soc 2015;63(9):1906–12. Available at: https://www.ncbi.nlm.nih.gov/pubmed/26312573. Accessed February 5, 2018.

29. Cooper C, Maxmin K, Selwood A, et al. The sensitivity and specificity of the modified conflict tactics scale for detecting clinically significant elder abuse. Int Psychogeriatr 2009;21(04):774.

30. Colby S, Ortman J. The baby boom cohort in the United States: 2012 to 2060 Population Estimates and Projections. Current population reports. 2014.

31. Dong X, Simon MA, Evans D. Elder self-neglect and hospitalization: findings from the Chicago health and aging project. J Am Geriatr Soc 2012;60(2):202–9.

32. Dong XQ. Elder abuse: systematic review and implications for practice. J Am Geriatr Soc 2015;63(6):1214–38.

33. Johannesen M, Logiudice D. Elder abuse: a systematic review of risk factors in community-dwelling elders. Age Ageing 2013;42(3):292–8.

34. Dong X, Chen R, Chang E, et al. Elder abuse and psychological well-being: a systematic review and implications for research and policy - a mini review. Gerontology 2013;59(2):132–42.

35. Kamavarapu Y, Ferriter M, Morton S, et al. Institutional abuse – characteristics of victims, perpetrators and organsations: a systematic review. Eur Psychiatry 2017;40:45–54.

36. Bows H. Practitioner views on the impacts, challenges, and barriers in supporting older survivors of sexual violence. Violence Against Women 2017. https://doi.org/10.1177/1077801217732348.

37. Burnes D, Henderson CR, Sheppard C, et al. Prevalence of financial fraud and scams among older adults in the United States: a systematic review and meta-analysis. Am J Public Health 2017 Aug;107(8):1295.

38. Laumann EO, Leitsch SA, Waite LJ. Elder mistreatment in the United States: prevalence estimates from a nation- ally representative study. J Gerontol B Psychol Sci Soc Sci 2008;63:S248–54.

39. Phelan A, Fealy G, Downes C. Piloting the older adult financial exploitation measure in adult safeguarding services. Arch Gerontol Geriatr 2017;70: 148–54.

40. Peterson JC, Burnes DP, Caccamise PL, et al. Financial exploitation of older adults: a population-based prevalence study. J Gen Intern Med 2014;29: 1615–23.

41. Wiglesworth A, Austin R, Corona M, et al. Bruising as a marker of physical elder abuse. J Am Geriatr Soc 2009;58:493–500.

42. Brozowski K, Hall DR. Aging and risk: physical and sexual abuse of elders in Canada. J Interpers Violence 2010;25(7):1183–99.

43. Rosen T, Lachs MS, Pillemer K. Sexual aggression between residents in nursing homes: literature synthesis of an underrecognized problem. J Am Geriatr Soc 2010;58(10):1970–9.

44. Teaster PB, Ramsey-Klawsnik H, Abner E, et al. Investigations of the sexual victimization of older women living in nursing homes. J Elder Abuse Negl 2015; 27(4–5):392–409.

45. Dong XQ. Medical implications of elder abuse and neglect. Clin Geriatr Med 2005;21(2):293–313.

46. Teaster PB, Roberto KA. The sexual abuse of older adults: APS cases and outcomes. Gerontologist 2004;44(6):788–96.

47. Beach SR, Schulz R, Castle NG, et al. Financial exploitation and psychological mistreatment among older adults: differences between African Americans and non-African Americans in a population-based survey. Gerontologist 2010. https://doi.org/10.1093/geront/gnq053. Accessed May 11, 2018.

48. Cadmus EO, Owoaje ET. Prevalence and correlates of elder abuse among older women in rural and urban communities in South Western Nigeria. Health Care Women Int 2012;33(10):973–84.

49. Schroeder M. Financial exploitation: when taking money amounts to elder abuse. US News and World Reports 2017.

50. Ramsey-Klawsnik H, Teaster PB, Mendiondo MS, et al. Sexual predators who target elders: findings from the first national study of sexual abuse in care facilities. J Elder Abuse Negl 2008;20(4):353–76.

51. Fraga S, Lindert J, Barros H, et al. Elder abuse and socioeconomic inequalities: a multilevel study in 7 European countries. Prev Med 2014;61:42–7.

52. Burnett J, Achenbaum W, Murphy K. Prevention and early identification of elder abuse. Clin Geriatr Med 2014;30(4):743–59.

53. Neale AV, Hwalek MA, Scott RO, et al. Validation of the Hwalek- Sengstock elder abuse screening test. J Appl Gerontol 1991;10(4):406–15. Reprinted by permission: Sage Publications, Thousand Oaks, CA.

54. Schofield MJ, Mishra GD. Validity of self-report screening scale for elder abuse: women's Health Australia Study. Gerontologist 2003;43(1):110–20.

55. Available at: http://eldermistreatment.usc.edu/wp-content/uploads/2016/10/Elder-Abuse-Screening-Tools-for-Healthcare-Professionals.pdf. Accessed May 11, 2018.

56. Naughton C, Drennan J, Lyons I, et al. Abuse and neglect of older people in Ireland (Report on the national study of elder abuse and neglect). Dublin (Republic of Ireland): National Centre for the Protection of Older People; 2010.

57. Ajomale O. Country report: ageing in Nigeria—current state, social and eco- nomic implications. African Gerontological Society; 2007. Available at: http://rcll-sociology-of-aging.org/system/files/Nigeria%202007_0.pdf. Accessed May 11, 2018.
58. Wiglesworth A. Screening for abuse and neglect of people with dementia. J Am Geriatr Soc 2010;58(3):493–500.
59. Dong X, Simon M, Mendes de Leon C, et al. Elder self-neglect and abuse and mortality risk in a community-dwelling population. J Am Med Assoc 2009; 302(5):517–26.
60. Available at: https://wallethub.com/edu/states-with-best-elder-abuse-protection/28754/. Accessed May 11, 2018.

Falls in the Geriatric Patient

Deborah J. Bolding, PhD[a], Ellen Corman, MRA[a,b],*

KEYWORDS

- Fall prevention • Older adults • Risk factors • Prevention

KEY POINTS

- Health professionals should encourage older adults to maintain health, active lifestyles and receive routine fall risk screening.
- Best practices for fall prevention are multifaceted, including medication management, home assessment and modification, and exercise for strength and balance.
- Older adults who adhere to fall prevention recommendations have fewer falls, fewer injurious falls, and use fewer paramedic and emergency department resources.
- Health professionals can reinforce adherence to fall prevention practices by supporting patients' commitment to change and encouraging them to develop a plan of action.

INTRODUCTION

Falls are the primary cause of injuries for older adults; can lead to decreased quality of life; and exact high individual, social, and health care costs. Careful assessment of individual fall risks and the provision of appropriate interventions, including treatment of coexisting medical conditions, medication review, exercise, and education about home and community safety, can lead to healthier aging.[1]

EPIDEMIOLOGY

Falls occur in approximately 25% of older adults aged 65 to 74 each year, and the rate increases to 29% for those in the 75 to 84 years category. For adults aged 85 and older, 36% are at risk for falling.[2] In the United States, falls in the older adult population contributed to 27,000 deaths, 2.8 million emergency department visits, and more than 80,000 hospitalizations.[2] Medical costs as a result of falls are estimated to be $50 billion annually, with Medicare and Medicaid paying $38 billion and $12 billion paid by private insurers and other payers.[3]

Disclosure Statement: There is no commercial relationship with direct financial interest in subject matter or materials discussed in the article for both authors.

[a] Trauma Service, Stanford Health Care, 300 Pasteur Drive, MC 5898, Stanford, CA 94305, USA;
[b] Injury Prevention and Community Engagement, Stanford Health Care/Stanford Medicine, Stanford, CA, USA
* Corresponding author. Trauma Service, Stanford Health Care, 300 Pasteur Drive, MC 5898, Stanford, CA 94305.
E-mail address: ecorman@stanfordhealthcare.org

Although falls occur at all ages, older adults are more vulnerable to injury after a fall, creating significant repercussions to health and independence. Older adults who sustain injurious falls are more likely to be discharged to a rehabilitation center or skilled nursing facility than younger adults and those who sustain one injurious fall are also at risk for subsequent injurious falls in the long term.[4,5] Expectations for full recovery following a severe fall injury are low. Older adults with hip fractures face a five to eight times increased risk of mortality during the first 3 months after the fracture, and are at risk for new functional mobility and self-care limitations, impaired balance, muscle weakness, low levels of physical activity, and further falls.[6] Sequelae of traumatic brain injury after a fall can include decreased independence in activities of daily living, cognitive and behavioral deficits, and the need for ongoing complex care for cognitive and motor deficits.[7]

FALL RISK FACTORS

Although the risk of falling becomes greater as one ages, many factors contribute to falls. Age alone should not determine interventions. Risk factors are categorized by whether or not they are intrinsic to the individual (eg, age, gender, cognitive deficits, chronic conditions), or extrinsic, or external to the individual (eg, medications, footwear, home environment).[8] History of falling is a strong independent risk factor for additional falls, particularly two or more falls in a 12-month period or an injurious fall.[9,10] Recent hospitalization is another predictor for increased fall risk, and it has been suggested that health care professionals do not provide adequate education programs to prevent falls in the posthospitalization recovery period.[11]

The World Health Organization suggested four categories for fall risk factors: (1) biologic, (2) behavioral, (3) environmental, and (4) socioeconomic.[12] This model is useful for reminding health care professionals that behavioral factors (eg, excess alcohol use, readiness to modify actions or environment), or socioeconomic risk factors (eg, inadequate housing or limited access to services) need to be addressed in conjunction with more traditional fall risk factors, such as number and type of medications and scores on balance tests (**Table 1**). Focus on individual risk factors may obscure broader areas and issues in which people need to be supported, such as housing, assistance with instrumental activities of daily living, and age-friendly environments.

Table 1 Fall risk factors	
Biologic	Age; race; gender; chronic illnesses (eg, neurologic diseases, arthritis, cancer); physical, sensory, cognitive, and affective declines
Behavioral	Multiple medications, lack of exercise, excess alcohol usage, inappropriate footwear, inattention, multitasking, hurrying
Environmental	Building design, insufficient lighting, slippery floors or surfaces, loose rugs, stairs, clutter, pets, uneven sidewalks or lack of paved walking areas, areas considered unsafe for walking for personal security reasons, lack of parks or inviting areas for walking or exercise
Socioeconomic	Inadequate housing, lack of social interaction, limited access to health and social services, lack of community resources, low income/education

Data from World Health Organization. WHO global report on falls prevention in older age. Available at: http://www.who.int/ageing/publications/Falls_prevention7March.pdf. Accessed April 8, 2018.

Biologic risk factors for falls include several illnesses and diseases that affect strength, range of motion, coordination, vision, hearing, balance, and endurance. Persons with neurologic disorders (eg, stroke, Parkinson disease, mild cognitive impairment, dementia, traumatic brain injury) have a higher rate of falls, as do persons with diabetes (with concomitant peripheral neuropathy or visual changes), cancer, orthopedic conditions, and decreased vision.[9,13] In persons with depressive symptoms, fall risk may be increased by 30%.[14] Fear of falling is another factor that contributes to increased fall risk, and often results from past falls.[15] Older adults with a fear of falling self-restrict their activities, possibly leading to additional falls and diminished quality of life.[15]

Classes of medications that increase the risk of falls include antidepressants, antihypertensives, diuretics, some analgesics, sedatives, and psychotropic medications.[16] The risk of falling is increased when new prescriptions are initiated, and with the use of two or more classes of fall-related drugs.[16,17] The complexity of mediating the balance between medications and falls is illustrated by the finding that although the use of antidepressants is associated with increased fall risk, the symptoms of depression (eg, lack of physical activity or awareness of the environment) are also risk factors for falling.

The rate of falling increases with the number of risk factors, increasing from a fall rate of 8% for older adults aged 75 and older with no fall risk factors to a 78% fall rate for those with four or more risk factors.[18] More positively, although many conditions are correlated with fall risk, the incidence of falls and injuries may be modified through education, medical or surgical intervention, environmental modifications, and exercise.

FALL RISK ASSESSMENT

The Centers for Disease Control and Prevention recommends that older adult patients always be asked about fall history, and has developed screening and referral guidelines for primary care physicians.[19] The Stopping Elderly Accidents, Deaths and Injuries (STEADI) Web site suggests that physicians routinely ask patients three questions: (1) "Have you fallen in the past year?" (2) "Do you feel unsteady when standing or walking?" and (3) "Do you worry about falling?" An affirmative to any of these questions indicates increased risk of falling and warrants further assessment for gait, strength, and balance.[19] The agency offers the STEADI Toolkit, with clinical practice guidelines, fall risk screening tools, and patient education and referral materials.[19]

Physical tests included in the STEADI are the 30-Second Chair Stand Test, which evaluates lower extremity strength, balance, and mobility; 4-Stage Balance; and Timed Up and Go. The STEADI algorithm recommends education and referrals for those patients in the highest risk categories, and a follow-up after 1 month to review the care plan and address barriers to adherence to a fall risk-reduction program.[19]

Other aspects of fall screening should consider vision, audition, cardiac factors (rate, rhythm, murmurs), depressive symptoms, fear of falling, and cognition.[14] When physical test scores are combined with other risk factors, such as comorbidities, medications, and previous falls, care providers can more readily identify patients that are at higher risk for falls and optimal interventions to meet the needs of individual patients.[14,20,21]

FALL PREVENTION INTERVENTIONS

Single and multifaceted fall prevention programs are associated with a lower risk of falls, especially when individualized for the patient.[22] The National Council on Aging

(NCOA) currently supports 13 evidence-based programs that meet the criteria for demonstrating effectiveness in reducing falls. Programs are individual or group-based and vary in frequency of delivery, costs for training leaders and delivering the program, and measured outcomes. Details of these programs are located on the NCOA Web site.[23]

Medications

Appropriate polypharmacy (use of five or more prescription drugs) has been defined as prescribing the correct medications under the appropriate circumstances to treat the right diseases.[17,24] It is estimated that 40% of older adults take five or more prescriptions, and this can lead to alterations in the pharmacokinetics, drug toxicities, and increased risk of falls.[25] In addition to understanding which medications place patients for the highest risk for falling, the physician, pharmacist, or nurse should ensure the patient (and family, if applicable) understands medication regimens (doses, times, administration methods), medication side effects including risk for falls, alcohol-drug interactions, and effects of over-the-counter medications and herbal products in combination with prescriptions (including over-the-counter medication sleep aids and melatonin).

Taking the medications at times that minimize waking at night to go to the bathroom or to avoid daytime drowsiness are important fall prevention considerations. Patients should be cautioned to observe for side effects that might lead to falls, particularly in the first few days after starting a new medication.

Vision

Visual changes in acuity, contrast sensitivity, visual fields, and depth perception are associated with increased fall risk.[26] Regular eye examinations are important in this population, because visual deficits can lead to decreased step accuracy, balance, and physical activity, and fear of falling.[26] Correction of visual problems (eg, surgery for cataracts, single-focus vs multifocal lenses) is possible in some cases, but if not, the patient should be referred to low vision services to incorporate mobility training, assistive device prescription and training, and environmental modifications at home and in the community.[26]

Vitamin D

Vitamin D deficiency is correlated with functional decline and muscle atrophy in older adults. However, evidence regarding the role of vitamin D in decreasing fall risk or the rate of falls has been contradictory.[27] A meta-analysis of 33 randomized trials found no association between calcium and vitamin D supplementation and the risk of hip and vertebral fractures in community-dwelling older adults.[28] This is in contrast to an additional meta-analysis that concluded vitamin D supplementation decreased the number of injurious falls and fractures.[22]

Exercise Programs for Active Older Adults

Health education and exercise are appropriate referrals for older adults who are at low risk for falls based on the STEADI screening and other factors. Patients should be encouraged to participate in individual or group exercise regimens to maintain or improve balance and strength, and to educate themselves about potential fall risks (eg, medication side effects and interactions and environmental hazards). The Centers for Disease Control and Prevention and NCOA have excellent education materials for older adults.[19,23,29] Spanish language education materials about exercise and activities are available from the National Institute on Aging (https://go4life.nia.nih.gov/spanish-resources) and NCOA, but resources for non-English speakers are limited.[23]

Community exercise programs designed for older adults are offered at senior centers, community centers, community colleges, YMCAs, and through private centers. Patients with Medicare Advantage Plans may have access to free fitness center programs, such as SilverSneakers (https://www.silversneakers.com/). Many YMCAs and senior centers offer an evidence-based fall prevention program called EnhanceFitness, which incorporates cardiovascular, strength, balance, and flexibility exercises.

Tai Chi training addresses postural control, flexibility, strength, balance, and coordination through a slow, rhythmic movement. Tai Chi-Moving for Better Balance is a center-based program that has been effective in improving fall risk measures.[30] Initial research about the benefits of Tai Chi was done with community-dwelling older adults, but subsequent studies reported benefits for frail older adults, including gains in strength and balance and decreased fear of falling.[31] Outcomes regarding the effect of Tai Chi on falls, particularly for older adults with a high risk of falling, has been mixed and it seems to be more effective for people with lower risk of falling.[31]

Many people do not like group education or exercise programs or gyms; classes may not fit their schedule or they may not have transportation or be able to afford the programs. Home-based programs that incorporate balance, strength, and flexibility exercises can achieve significant reduction in rate of falls and risk of falling; however, older adults often identify walking as their primary form of exercise. Although brisk walking is an excellent form of exercise for helping patients manage a variety of health conditions, improve mood, and strengthening, walking alone is not sufficient for maintaining or improving balance and reducing the rate of falls.[32] Balance exercises can supplement a walking program, particularly in climates where temperatures and conditions limit outdoor activities.

Exercise Programs for At-Risk Older Adults

For persons who are at higher risk for falls (eg, past falls, health conditions, frailty, medications, postoperative, using mobility aids, fear of falling, depressive symptoms), education should be focused on individual fall risk factors and how to modify risks through exercise and behavioral and environmental changes. Patients should be encouraged to develop a plan of action, and referrals for physical therapy and occupational therapy, vision and hearing screening, community-based falls prevention programs, and community-based exercise programs are often indicated.

The Otago Exercise Program (OEP) is a strength and exercise program that was designed as a home-based program for frail elderly with the highest risk for falling. Initial and subsequent randomized controlled trials reported as much as a 35% reduction in falls.[33] The program is taught in six sessions over a period of 1 year by physical or occupational therapists or nurses, with telephone follow-up between sessions, and advanced as the patients' balance and strength improve. Participation in the OEP has been shown to improve performance on the Timed Up and Go, 30-Second Chair Stand, and Four Stage Balance test, and actually reduce the risk of death and the rate of falls over a 1-year period.[34,35] The OEP has been adapted for teaching in physical therapy clinics, in groups for older adults who have mild balance problems, and with other types of exercises, with outcomes similar to the home-based instruction.[34]

The benefits of exercise for health at all ages is well documented, and older adults should be encouraged to participate. Exercise programs alone, however, may not be enough to reduce the risk of serious fall injuries in sedentary older adults. The next section discusses more comprehensive interventions.

Multiple Interventions and Multifactorial Programs

Multiple intervention programs typically include standardized education and interventions delivered to all participants in the group, whereas participants in multifactorial programs receive individualized assessment and interventions based on personal risk factors.[32] Insurance providers, health care institutions, senior centers, and community centers among others offer a variety of multiple intervention programs for their constituents. Local offerings are readily found via Internet search for "fall prevention classes in [city name]." Education programs may be led by health educators, occupational therapists, physical therapists, nurses, physicians, other fitness professionals, or by lay leaders. Educational programs seem to be most effective when combined with exercise, home safety, and vision assessment.[32] Outcome data for community programs are not always available or may only be reported internally to the organization sponsoring the program.

One multiple intervention program that has demonstrated efficacy in reducing falls, emergency room visits, and hospitalizations is the Healthy Steps for Older Adults program.[23] The program consists of two 2-hour sessions covering a wide range of topics including environmental safety, exercises, nutrition, foot health, sensory deficits, medication, health and substance use, active lifestyles, social connectedness, and mental and spiritual well-being. Health care savings were estimated at $840 per person over 12 months for Healthy Steps for Older Adults participants when compared with a group of nonparticipants.[36]

Two programs that have been adopted nationally are A Matter of Balance (AMOB) and Stepping On. Both programs meet for eight 2-hour sessions and have demonstrated efficacy in reducing falls. AMOB, the more widely disseminated program, is taught by lay leaders (coaches).[37] Through facilitated discussions in AMOB sessions, participants learn practical strategies for increasing the safety of their environment and decreasing fear of falling. They set goals to increase activity and learn exercises for strength and balance, improved falls efficacy, improved balance, strength, and mobility measures. Because this is a lay-led model, the comparatively low cost of providing this program makes AMOB an economical choice. Participation was associated with cost savings in unplanned inpatient, skilled nursing facility, and home health settings in the year following the program, reducing medical costs by an estimated $938 per year.[37,38]

Stepping On, which has demonstrated a 31% decrease in falls, meets for seven 2-hour sessions, followed by an additional session 3 months after the initial classes.[39] Guest speakers include a physical therapist (for three visits), pharmacist, vision expert, and community safety expert. A home visit to consider home safety concerns and to answer other questions is also offered to participants. Stepping On results in a $134 net benefit per participant.[23] **Table 2** provides more information about cost savings across different programs.

Home and Community Safety

The premise of home safety assessment and modification is that a safe home environment makes falls less likely. There is evidence that home safety assessments reduce the rate and risk for falling, although effectiveness is greater for persons with a history of falls and a higher number of risk factors.[32] Comprehensive functional assessment of participants in their homes seems to be more effective than using a screening checklist, particularly when services are provided by an occupational therapist.[32] Occupational therapy and physical therapy home-based interventions for environmental modifications, safe performance, problem-solving, energy conservation, fall recovery,

Table 2
Comparison of evidence-based, community-based programs

A Matter of Balance	Otago Exercise Program	Stepping On	Tai Chi: Moving for Better Balance
8-session workshop to reduce fear of falling and increase activity among older adults in the community	Individual program of muscle strengthening and balance exercises prescribed by a physical therapist for frail older adults living at home (aged 80+)	7-wk program (plus follow-up and home visit) offers older adults living in the community proven strategies to reduce falls and increase self-confidence	Balance and gait training program of controlled movement for older adults and people with balance disorders
• 97% of participants feel more comfortable talking about their fear of falling	• 35% reduction in falls rate	• 30% reduction in falls rate	• 55% reduction in falls rate
• 99% of participants plan to continue exercising	• $429 net benefit per participant	• $134 net benefit per participant	• $530 net benefit per participant
• $938 savings in unplanned medical costs per Medicare beneficiary	• 127% ROI	• 64% ROI	• $509% ROI

Abbreviation: ROI, return on investment.

Data from Carande-Kulis V, Stevens J, Florence C, et al. A cost-benefit analysis of three older adult falls prevention interventions. J Safety Res 2015;52:65–70; and Report to Congress in November 2013: the Centers for Medicare & Medicaid Services evaluation of community-based wellness and prevention programs under section 4202(b) of the Affordable Care Act. Available at: http://innovation.cms.gov/Files/reports/Community WellnessRTC.pdf; and *Adapted from* National Council on Aging. Evidence-based falls prevention programs: saving lives, saving money. Available at: https://www.ncoa.org/resources/falls-prevention-programs-saving-lives-saving-money-infographic-3/. Accessed April 8, 2018; with permission.

and exercise can result in wide-ranging improvement in older adults, including areas of instrumental activities of daily living and activities of daily living, confidence, decreased fear of falling, and use of adaptive strategies.[40]

The Community Aging in Place – Advancing Better Living for Elders model is a patient-directed, 5-month program that combines services from an occupational therapist (six visits); nurse (four visits); and 1 day's work from a maintenance/handy person to provide home safety modifications, install assistive devices, and provide basic home repairs.[41] Common home modification services include installing railings and grab bars, nonskid treads or mats, improving lighting, repairing floors, raising toilet seats, and installing flexible shower hoses and doorbells. Preliminary findings with the first 100 participants demonstrated improvement in the areas of function, home hazards, and depressive symptoms.[41]

Behavioral Aspects of Fall Prevention

The previous sections described interventions that have been found to be effective in reducing the risks and rate of falls for older adults, with concomitant social and economic savings. The interventions are designed to improve the knowledge, skills, attitudes, and behaviors of older adults related to fall prevention. The underlying assumption in this medical framework is that older adults view the risks similarly to health professionals and are ready to be "educated." If not, health professionals are responsible for trying to motivate and persuade them. If older adults elect to not make changes, they may be viewed as lacking self-awareness, minimizing and denying risk factors, or noncompliant.

This model is not an optimal framework for eliciting behavioral change. The identification of fall risks and recommendations for behavioral changes creates other risks for older adults, such as fear of dependence, and the loss of identity, dignity, and meaningful goals and activities.[42] Older adults may reject recommendations that are inconvenient, unwelcome, or not seen as relevant (eg, that is good advice for "older" people, but not them).[43,44] These factors also explain limited adherence with exercise, home modifications, and other recommendations by health professionals.

Other barriers to participation in exercise, fall prevention classes, or changes in the environment include lack of transportation, financial resources, and cognitive or physical abilities to participate in community-based programs. Lower participation in fall prevention programs has been observed in persons with less education; those living in disadvantaged areas; and those classified as obese, with fair or poor self-reported health, and who had problems walking.[45] There are multiple options for addressing these problems. Older adults who are unable to attend community-based programs for health or other reasons can be taught home-based exercise programs or use DVDs or online applications to promote better balance and reduce fall risks. Health professionals can work with family, caregivers, or case managers to refer families to individual resources.

To improve adherence to balance activities, or for persons who do not like exercise or group programs, an approach such as the Lifestyle Integrated Functional Exercise may be appropriate. It delivers balance and strength exercises by concentrating on everyday activities as triggers for the exercises.[46] For example, older adults might practice one leg stand exercises while brushing their teeth, or leg strengthening exercises while bending to retrieve objects from the floor or a lower cabinet. The Lifestyle Integrated Functional Exercise program demonstrated a 31% reduction in the rate of falls, and has been adapted for group settings, although outcomes for the group model are not yet known.[46,47]

The reasons for nonadherence, and methods for healthier behaviors, are critical because older adults who adhere to fall prevention recommendations have been found to have fewer falls, fewer injurious falls, and used fewer paramedic and emergency department resources.[48] The Transtheoretical Model and Stages of Change can help health professionals understand older adults' readiness for change.[48] Persons who are in the precontemplation and contemplation stages of change do not intend to take any immediate actions, perhaps because they are not informed about the issues, or perhaps because the programs offered do not meet their needs. In this stage, health care providers might provide support for existing positive fall prevention actions (eg, taking medications correctly, taking vitamin D), and provide education about the pros and cons of acting.

In the preparation stage, the person is ready to make a change and develop a plan of action. This is the stage in which older adults might decide to enroll in exercise classes or fall prevention programs. Providing them with information about local resources might reinforce their decision to change. Persons who are in the action stage have modified their behaviors to reduce fall risks and rate and should be supported in continuing their positive behaviors through this stage and the maintenance stage.

Adherence to recommended behavioral change is also influenced by the patient-caregiver relationship. Patients who perceive that doctors know them as individuals more consistently follow treatment plans. Collaboration and demonstrating warmth, openness, and interest further enhances adherence.[49] Motivational interviewing, which focuses on helping patients identify and resolve ambivalence about behavior change, builds on a good working relationship between the patient and health care provider. A specific direction for change is discussed, then the patient's ideas and feelings are elicited, validated, and reinforced. In the planning phase, the patient and care provider develop a commitment to change and plan of action, with a focus on eliciting the patient's ideas about solutions.[50]

Although there are several models that might be useful for understanding behavioral change, two others are discussed here. Social Cognitive Theory considers how perceived control over learning, or perceived self-efficacy, is developed through achievement, vicarious learning, social support and reinforcement, and emotional arousal. These factors contribute to initiating and continuing healthy behaviors.[51] A second model, the Theory of Planned Behavior, describes how the intention to perform a behavior is influenced by one's attitude about the intervention, subjective norms relative to the activity, and one's perceived control (or self-efficacy) over the change process.[52] These theories are useful for guiding interventions. For example, a person with low self-efficacy for preventing falls might not believe an exercise program could help them. Establishing small, achievable exercise goals could lead to improved self-efficacy and intention to continue the program. Participating in a group program, such as AMOB, where participants discuss their plans for change, and their successes, might change one's normative beliefs, thus increasing the likelihood for making behavioral changes.

SUMMARY

Falls in older adults are caused by a complex interplay of biologic, behavioral, environmental, and socioeconomic risk factors. Prevention of falls continues to be an elusive goal: every 11 seconds an older adult is treated in the emergency room for a fall; and every 19 minutes, an older adult dies from a fall.[23] With 10,000 people turning 65 each day, it is imperative that those at the highest risk receive interventions to decrease the risk and rate of falls, and that those at lower risk be educated about maintaining healthy lifestyles.[53]

REFERENCES

1. Rubenstein LZ. Falls in older people: epidemiology, risk factors and strategies for prevention. Age Ageing 2006;35:ii37–41.
2. Bergen G, Stevens MR, Burns ER. Falls and fall injuries among adults aged (greater or equal to) 65 years—United States, 2014. MMWR Morb Mortal Wkly Rep 2016;65:993–8.
3. Florence CS, Bergen G, Atherly A, et al. Medical costs of fatal and nonfatal falls in older adults. J Am Geriatr Soc 2018;66(4):693–8. Available at: https://onlinelibrary.wiley.com/doi/abs/10.1111/jgs.15304.
4. James MK, Victor MC, Saghir SM, et al. Characterization of fall patients: does age matter? J Safety Res 2018;64:83–92.
5. Pohl P, Nordin E, Lundquist A. Community-dwelling older people with an injurious fall are likely to sustain new injurious falls within 5 years: a prospective long-term follow-up study. BMC Geriatr 2014;14:120.
6. Haentjens P, Magaziner J, Colo'n-Emric CS, et al. Meta-analysis: excess mortality after hip fracture among older women and men. Ann Intern Med 2010;152:380–90.

7. Mas MF, Mathews A, Gilbert-Baffoe E. Rehabilitation needs of the elder with traumatic brain injury. Phys Med Rehabil Clin N Am 2017;28:829–42.

8. Gale CR, Cooper C, Sayer AA. Prevalence and risk factors for falls in older men and women: the English longitudinal study of ageing. Age Ageing 2016;45: 789–94.

9. Ambrose AF, Paul G, Hausdorff JM. Risk factors for falls among older adults: a review of the literature. Maturitas 2013;75:51–61.

10. Deandrea S, Lucenteforte E, Bravi F, et al. Risk factors for falls in community-dwelling older people: a systematic review and meta-analysis. Epidemiology 2010;21(5):658–68.

11. Hill A, Hoffman T, Beer C, et al. Falls after discharge from hospital: is there a gap between older peoples' knowledge about falls prevention strategies and the research evidence? Gerontologist 2011;51:653–62.

12. World Health Organization. WHO global report on falls prevention in older age. Available at: http://www.who.int/mediacentre/factsheets/fs344/en/. Accessed April 14, 2018.

13. Gopinath B, McMahon CM, Burlutsky, et al. Hearing and vision impairment and the 5-year incidence of falls in older adults. Age Ageing 2016;45:409–14.

14. Hoffman GJ, Hays RD, Wallace SP, et al. Depressive symptomatology and fall risk among community-dwelling older adults. Soc Sci Med 2017;178:206–33.

15. Jorstad EC, Hauer K, Becker C, et al. Measuring the psychological outcomes of falling: a systematic review. J Am Geriatr Soc 2005;53:501–10.

16. Musich S, Want SS, Ruiz J, et al. Falls-related drug use and risk of falls among older adults: a study in a US Medicare population. Drugs Aging 2017;34:555–65.

17. Zia A, Kamaruzzaman SB, Tan MP. The consumption of two or more fall risk-increasing drugs rather than polypharmacy is associated with falls. Geriatr Gerontol Int 2017;17:463–70.

18. Tinetti M, Speechley M, Ginter SF. Risk factors for falls among elderly persons living in the community. N Engl J Med 1988;319:1701–7.

19. Centers for Disease Control (CDC). STEADI (stopping elderly accidents, deaths, & injuries). Available at: https://www.cdc.gov/steadi/index.html. Accessed April 13, 2018.

20. Hallford DJ, Nicholson G, Sanders K, et al. The association between anxiety and falls: a meta-analysis. J Gerontol B Psychol Sci Soc Sci 2016;72:729–41.

21. Khow KSF, Visvanathan R. Falls in the aging population. Clin Geriatr Med 2017; 33:357–68.

22. Tricco AC, Thomas SM, Veroniki AA, et al. Comparisons of interventions for preventing falls in older adults: a systematic review and meta-analysis. JAMA 2017; 318(17):1687–99.

23. National Council on Aging. Falls prevention: keeping older adults safe and active. 2018. Available at: https://www.ncoa.org/healthy-aging/falls-prevention/. Accessed April 8, 2018.

24. Cooper JA, Cadogan CA, Patterson SM, et al. Interventions to improve the appropriate use of polypharmacy in older people: a Cochrane systematic review. BMJ Open 2015;5:e009235.

25. Park H, Satoh H, Miki A. Medications associated with falls in older people: systematic review of publications from a recent 5-year period. Eur J Clin Pharmacol 2015;71:1429–40.

26. Blaylock SE, Vogtle LK. Falls prevention interventions for older adults with low vision: a scoping review. Can J Occup Ther 2017;84:139–47.

27. De Jongh RT, van Schoor NM, Lips P. Changes in vitamin D endocrinology during aging in adults. Mol Cell Endocrinol 2017;453:144–50.

28. Zhao J, Zeng X, Wang J, et al. Association between calcium or vitamin D supplementation and fracture incidence in community-dwelling older adults: a systematic review and meta-analysis. JAMA 2017;318:2466–82.

29. National Institute on Aging at the NIH. Great! You're on your way to a healthier you. 2018. Available at: https://go4life.nia.nih.gov/get-started. Accessed April 8, 2018.

30. Li F, Harmer P, Glasgow R. Translation of an effective Tai Chi intervention into a community-based falls-prevention program. Am J Public Health 2008;98(7):1195–8.

31. Hackney ME, Wolf SL. Impact of Tai Chi Chu'an practice on balance and mobility in older adults: an integrative review of 20 years of research. J Geriatr Phys Ther 2014;37:127–35.

32. Gillespie LD, Robertson MC, Gillespie WJ, et al. Interventions for preventing falls in older people living in the community. Cochrane Database Syst Rev 2012;(2):CD007146.

33. Campbell AJ, Robertson MC. Comprehensive approach to fall prevention on a national level. Clin Geriatr Med 2010;26:719–31.

34. Shubert TE, Smith ML, Jiang L, et al. Disseminating the Otago exercise program in the United States: perceived and actual physical performance improvements from participants. J Appl Gerontol 2018;37(1):79–98.

35. Thomas S, Mackintosh S, Halbert J. Does the "Otago exercise programme" reduce mortality and falls in older adults?: a systematic review and meta-analysis. Age Ageing 2010;39(6):681–7.

36. Albert SM, Raviotta J, Lin CJ, et al. Cost-effectiveness of a statewide falls prevention program in Pennsylvania: healthy steps for older adults. Am J Manag Care 2016;22:638–44.

37. Smith ML, Jiang L, Ory MG. Falls efficacy among older adults enrolled in an evidence-based program to reduce fall-related risk. Fam Community Health 2012;35:256–63.

38. Report to Congress: the Centers for Medicare & Medicaid Services' evaluation of community-based wellness and prevention programs under section 4202 (b) of the Affordable Care Act. Available at: https://innovation.cms.gov/Files/reports/CommunityWellnessRTC.pdf. Accessed April 8, 2018.

39. Clemson L, Cumming RG, Kendig H, et al. The effectiveness of a community-based program for reducing the incidence of falls in the elderly: a randomized trial. J Am Geriatr Soc 2004;52:1487–94.

40. Gitlin LN, Winter L, Dennis MP, et al. A randomized trial of a multicomponent home intervention to reduce functional difficulties in older adults. J Am Geriatr Soc 2006;54:809–16.

41. Szanton SL, Wolf JL, Leff B, et al. Preliminary data from community aging in place, advancing better living for elders, a patient-directed team-based intervention to improve physical function and decrease nursing home utilization. J Am Geriatr Soc 2015;63:371–4.

42. Rudman D, Egan MY, McGrath CE. Low vision rehabilitation, age-related vision loss, and risk: a critical interpretive synthesis. Gerontologist 2016;56:e32–45.

43. Mikolaizak AS, Lord SR, Tiedemann A, et al. Adherence to a multifactorial fall prevention program following paramedic care: predictors and impact on falls and health service use. Results from an RCT a priori subgroup analysis. Australas J Ageing 2018;37:54–61.

44. Yardley L, Donovan-Hall M, Francis K, et al. Older people's views of advice about falls prevention: a qualitative study. Health Educ Res 2006;21:508–17.

45. Meron D, Pye V, Macniven R, et al. Prevalence and correlates of participation in fall prevention exercise/physical activity by older adults. Prev Med 2012;55: 613–7.

46. Clemson L, Singh MAF, Bundy A, et al. Integration of balance and strength training into daily life activity to reduce rate of falls in older people (the LiFE study): randomised parallel trial. BMJ 2012;345:14.

47. Fleig L, McAllister MM, Chen P, et al. Health behavior change theory meets falls prevention: feasibility of a habit-based balance and strength exercise intervention for older adults. Psychol Sport Exerc 2016;22:114–22.

48. Prochaska JO, Redding CA, Evers KE. The transtheoretical model and stages of social change. In: Glanz K, Rimer K, Viswanath K, editors. Health behavior: theory, research, and practice. Hoboken (NJ): John Wiley and Sons; 2015. p. 125–48.

49. Duggan A, Street RL Jr. Interpersonal communication in health and illness. In: Glanz K, Rimer K, Viswanath K, editors. Health behavior: theory, research, and practice. Hoboken (NJ): John Wiley and Sons; 2015. p. 243–67.

50. Elwyn G, Dehlendorf C, Epstein RM, et al. Shared decision making and motivational interviewing: achieving patient-centered care across the spectrum of health care problems. Ann Fam Med 2014;12:270–5.

51. Kelder SH, Hoelscher D. How individuals, environments and health behaviors interact: social cognitive theory. In: Glanz K, Rimer K, Viswanath K, editors. Health behavior: theory, research, and practice. Hoboken (NJ): John Wiley and Sons; 2015. p. 159–83.

52. Montaño DE, Kasprzyk D. Theory of reasoned action, theory of planned behavior, and the integrated behavioral model. In: Glanz K, Rimer K, Viswanath K, editors. Health behavior: theory, research, and practice. Hoboken (NJ): John Wiley and Sons; 2015. p. 95–124.

53. Kulinski K, DiCocco C, Skowronski S, et al. Advancing community-based falls prevention programs for older adults: the work of the administration for community living/administration. Front Public Health 2017;5:1–5.

Driving in the Geriatric Population

Wendy R. Greene, MD[a],*, Randi Smith, MD[b]

KEYWORDS

- Distracted driving • Geriatric • Elderly • Motorvehicle crash • Motor vehicle collision

KEY POINTS

- The older adult is susceptible to injury and has an increased risk of involvement in a motor vehicle crash despite seat belt use and lack of impaired driving.
- In 2015, more than 6800 older adults were killed and more than 260,000 were treated in emergency departments for motor vehicle crash injuries.
- The perfect storm of aging drivers and increasing morbidity and mortality associated with motor vehicle crashes is of utmost importance to study and prevent.

The significant decline in motor vehicle injury has been one of the most promising public health initiatives in this century. A concerted effort to decrease fatalities per million miles traveled was due to a combination of safer vehicles, safer roadways, and driver awareness. Unfortunately, despite these advances, the older population aged 65 and older are more likely to die or be severely injured. In 2015, more than 6800 older adults were killed and more than 260,000 were treated in emergency departments for motor vehicle crash injuries. The daily rates of elderly crash related deaths and injuries are 19 and 712 respectively.[1] These daunting statistics has prompted the Eastern Association of Surgery for Trauma (EAST) to query and publish on this topic. Furthermore, as the aging population increases, so does the number of licensed drivers. There were more than 40 million licensed older drivers in 2015, which is a 50% increase from 1999.[2,3] The perfect storm of aging drivers and increasing morbidity and mortality associated with motor vehicle crashes is of utmost importance to study and prevent.

The older adult is susceptible to injury and has an increased risk of involvement in a motor vehicle crash despite seat belt use and lack of impaired driving.

Disclosure: The authors have nothing to disclose.
[a] Emory University Department of Surgery, 1365 Clifton Road NE Building A, 4th floor, Atlanta, GA 30322, USA; [b] Emory University School of Medicine, Grady Hospital, 80 Jesse Hill Jr. Drive Southeast, Atlanta, GA 30303, USA
* Corresponding author. 1241 Zimmer Drive Northeast, Atlanta GA 30306.
E-mail address: wendy.ricketts.greene@emory.edu

WHO IS MOST AT RISK?

- Involvement in fatal crashes, per mile traveled, begins increasing among drivers aged 70 to 74 and are highest among drivers aged 85 and older. This trend has been attributed more to an increased susceptibility to injury and medical complications among older drivers rather than an increased risk of crash involvement.[4]
- Across all age groups, men have substantially higher death rates than women.[4]
- Age-related declines in vision and cognitive functioning (ability to reason and remember), as well as physical changes, may affect some older adults' driving abilities.[5]

Consider the older driver and what factors may put them at increased risk for being involved and sustaining injury during a crash. The comorbidities, frailty, decline in visual, auditory, and motor function found in this population can be contributing factors. The older population who is disproportionately plagued with dementia can experience delayed neurologic response times while driving. The delayed response times and declines in vision can lead to an inability to time turns with oncoming traffic as well as transition between acceleration versus braking. The auditory cues needed for yielding to an emergency vehicle and avoiding an impending danger are hampered by hearing loss in the older driver. In addition, an altered mental status may be an acquired condition due to lower cerebral perfusion after changes in the dose of antihypertensive medications or due to hypoglycemia. Unfortunately, the older driver is often prescribed multiple medications that can have various interactions that effect cognition and reactions that are not recognized until an injury occurs.

HOW CAN OLDER DRIVER DEATHS AND INJURIES BE PREVENTED?

Older adults take several steps to stay safe while driving.

- High incidence of seat belt use
  Although 60% of passenger vehicle occupants (drivers and passengers) aged 65 to 74 and 71% of passenger vehicle occupants aged 75+ killed in crashes were wearing seat belts at the time of the crash, seat belt use among younger adults ranged from 37% (among those aged 21–24) to 54% (among those aged 55–64).[6]
- Tendency to drive when environmental factors are optimal for reducing the risk of injury
  Older drivers tend to limit their driving during inclement weather, in the dark, and on high-speed roads, in comparison to younger drivers.[7]
- Lower incidence of impaired driving
  Older adult drivers are less likely to drive while intoxicated compared with younger drivers.[8] In 2015, only 6% of drivers older than 75 who were involved in fatal crashes had a blood alcohol concentration (BAC) of 0.08 g/dL or higher, compared with 28% of drivers aged 21 to 24 years. Overall, 20% of all drivers involved in fatal crashes had a BAC of 0.08 g/dL or higher.[9]

Despite advances in automotive design, elderly front seat passengers are at greater risk for injury when compared with younger passengers. Geriatric drivers sustain more injuries related to air bag deployment. In addition, lap and shoulder belts may contribute to injuries. These injuries are the result of the restraint device not being positioned properly due to the higher incidence of kyphoscoliosis with aging.[10]

Injuries are also reduced for rear seat passengers with a properly placed seat belt. Unrestrained drivers and occupants are obviously at increased risk for injuries. Studies support behavior modification, and use of reminders to encourage seat belt use can increase compliance and protection from most injuries. It must be remembered that although restraint devices save lives, lap belts are known to increase the incidence of hollow viscus injury.

Elderly drivers avoid driving in urban areas, during heavy traffic times, or at night. Despite their behavior modification, Renner and colleagues[11] reported that the elderly have a higher rate of collisions resulting in injuries during the early evening hours when compared with younger drivers. The reason for the increased crash-related injuries has been attributed to diminished motor and sensory functions during the evening hours when the elderly experience "sun downing."

With the knowledge that the elderly have the highest mortality of any age group when involved in a motor vehicle crash (MVC), it is important to reduce MVC-related mortality. One of the ways is to decrease the pedestrian versus auto-related injuries. Studies have demonstrated that elderly pedestrians struck by a vehicle accounted for most of the deaths for this mechanism of injury. Fortunately, Lyons and colleagues[12] were able to demonstrate that traffic-calming measures can be implemented to combat pedestrian injuries and decrease fatalities among all age groups.

The environmental and behavioral interventions for elderly do not necessarily prevent vehicle-related injuries, and legislation has been shown to be beneficial initially but does not have a sustained effect. Because elderly drivers self-restrict at different ages for different reasons, it is difficult to apply universal driver restrictions because not all older drivers need to have a restricted license. Many factors can contribute to needs for driver restrictions, besides age. These factors include sun downing, visual audio impairments, and delayed response times. Research shows that cessation of driving in seniors can lead to depression and loss of independence. When seniors drive less, they fall into the low mileage bias. Arrhythmias are known to increase the risk of a crash when compared with visual or hearing impairment. Diabetic drivers with coronary artery disease (CAD) are at an increased risk for crashing with a subsequent injury.

MVCs frequently occur at intersections at low speeds because elders have difficulty in rapid maneuvers. Some studies support that dynamic visual acuity should be tested rather than the static testing that is used in most licensing agencies. Current screening tools are not effective in determining at-risk drivers.

The lower incidence of impaired driving in the older population compared with younger drivers is known to reduce the incidence of accidents. It is well established that alcohol and/or drug intoxication significantly increases the risk of being involved in an MVC. The elderly may be even more sensitive to the effects of drugs and alcohol than their younger counterparts because of age-related derangements in metabolism, comorbid medical conditions, and medication interactions.[10]

Based on the EAST evidence-based review of geriatric trauma, significant recommendations were made to address injury prevention in the older driver.[10]

The recommendations are as follows:

CAR ENGINEERING ADVANCEMENTS

Ongoing engineering advancements in car safety restraint systems should take into account passenger-specific factors, such as age, weight, and height. The current safety restraint standards for vehicles do not take into account the vulnerability to injury of the elderly. In low-speed collisions, the very restraint systems designed to prevent injury may be contributing to chest/torso injuries in the elderly. An ideal solution would entail the development and implementation of sex-, height-, and weight-sensitive restraints.

ENVIRONMENTAL OR BEHAVIORAL INTERVENTIONS

Seat belt reminder signs should be placed at exit points in areas with significant numbers of senior drivers, such as senior centers or assisted living facilities. Furthermore, pedestrian crosswalks should be marked with stop signs or traffic lights. Traffic-calming measures should be installed be in areas of high pedestrian density. The elderly pedestrian is at high risk of injury when struck by a vehicle. However, it seems that crosswalks without stop signs or traffic lights are associated with an increased risk for injury. Pedestrians may consider a crosswalk to be safe simply because it is a crosswalk, without considering driver cues or behaviors. In addition, lowering speeds and adding speed bumps or traffic circles in heavily traveled areas were associated with fewer fatal pedestrian crashes. These environmental and behavioral interventions should be considered but may also have important implications for businesses and residents.

RISK SCREENING STRATEGIES

The elderly should be screened for alcohol abuse, frailty, diabetes, hearing impairments, visual impairments, and CAD if they are continuing to drive because these conditions are known to increase the risk for MVC-related injuries. Behavioral interventions to prevent MVC-related injury have been shown to be effective for elderly drivers. These types of programs aim to change elderly driver behaviors to enhance their safety and reduce injury. Seat belt awareness programs can be successful in changing the habits of a generation that grew up without mandatory seat belt legislation. However, the research on other behavioral interventions is lacking. There is a need for additional direct intervention investigations. Risk reduction strategies strive to identify key risk factors that place elderly drivers at higher risk for MVCs and injury. Several medical conditions, such as arrhythmias, CAD, diabetes, and hearing impairment, have been implicated. Universal screening for alcohol and drug use causing driving impairment, irrespective of age, should be a goal. Finally, frailty has been increasingly found to be associated with injury outcomes. A frailty assessment may be a useful tool to help identify at-risk aging drivers, and its predictive ability should be prospectively studied. It must be noted that the elderly driver population is heterogeneous; thus, any generalized limitation on driving privileges based on medical conditions is not indicated, and individual patients should be screened for significant impairments that might affect their ability to drive safely.

SUMMARY

In summary, the paucity of controlled studies in the area of motor vehicle–related injury prevention among the elderly demonstrates a significant information gap; further research is needed to strengthen future evidence-based guidelines and to influence preventative health strategies for seniors.

REFERENCES

1. Centers for Disease Control and Prevention, National Center for Injury Prevention and Control. Web-based injury statistics query and reporting system (WISQARS). Atlanta (GA): CDC; 2017. Available at: https://www.cdc.gov/injury/wisqars/index.html. Accessed November 29, 2017.
2. Federal Highway Administration, Department of Transportation (US). Highway statistics 2015. Washington, DC: FHWA; 2016. Available at: https://www.fhwa.

dot.gov/policyinformation/statistics/2015/dl20.cfm. Accessed December 21, 2016.
3. Federal Highway Administration, Department of Transportation (US). Highway statistics 2015. Washington, DC: FHWA. Available at: https://www.fhwa.dot.gov/policyinformation/statistics/2015/dl20.cfm. Accessed October 3, 2018.
4. Insurance Institute for Highway Safety (IIHS). Fatality facts 2015, older people. Arlington (VA): IIHS; 2016. Available at: http://www.iihs.org/iihs/topics/t/older-drivers/fatalityfacts/older-people/2015. Accessed December 21, 2016.
5. Owsley C. Driver capabilities in transportation in an aging society: a decade of experience. technical papers and reports from a Conference: Bethesda, MD; Nov. 7–9, 1999. Washington, DC: Transportation Research Board; 2004.
6. National Highway Safety Traffic Administration, Department of Transportation (US). Traffic safety facts 2015: a compilation of motor vehicle crash data from the fatality analysis reporting system and the general estimates system. Washington, DC: NHTSA; 2017. Available at: https://crashstats.nhtsa.dot.gov/Api/Public/Publication/812384. Accessed November 13, 2017.
7. Naumann RB, Dellinger AM, Kresnow MJ. Driving self-restriction in high-risk conditions: how do older drivers compare to others? J Safety Res 2011;42:67–71.
8. Quinlan KP, Brewer RD, Siegel P, et al. Alcohol–impaired driving among U.S. adults: 1993–2002. Am J Prev Med 2005;28:346–50.
9. National Highway Traffic Safety Administration, Department of Transportation (US). Alcohol-impaired driving, 2015 data. Washington, DC: NHTSA; 2016. Available at: https://crashstats.nhtsa.dot.gov/Api/Public/ViewPublication/812350. Accessed December 21, 2016.
10. Crandall M, Streams J, Duncan T, et al. Motor vehicle collision–related injuries in the elderly: an eastern association for the surgery of trauma evidence-based review of risk factors and prevention. J Trauma Acute Care Surg 2015;79(1):152–8.
11. Renner CH, Heldt KA, Swegle JR. Diurnal variation and injury due to motor vehicle crashes in older trauma patients. Traffic Inj Prev 2011;12(6):593Y598.
12. Lyons RA, Jones SJ, Newcombe RG, et al. The influence of local politicians on pedestrian safety. Inj Prev 2006;12(5):312Y315.

Suicide in the Elderly
A Multidisciplinary Approach to Prevention

Steven E. Brooks, MD[a], Sigrid K. Burruss, MD[b],
Kaushik Mukherjee, MD, MSCI[b],*

KEYWORDS

- Elderly • Geriatric • Suicide • Prevention • Risk factors • Multidisciplinary
- Telehealth • Physician extender

KEY POINTS

- Suicide in the elderly is a growing public health problem worldwide, resulting in significant mortality and family turmoil.
- Elderly patients are at dramatically increased risk of suicide compared with younger individuals.
- Numerous risk factors for suicide include mental illness, physical illness, family, financial, insurance, and social factors.
- Firearms significantly increase the likelihood of successful suicide, and firearms interventions may help to save lives.
- A multidisciplinary, community-based approach involving initial screening interventions with referral to mental health professionals and subsequent follow-up and telehealth interventions may comprise a future approach to this vulnerable population.

INTRODUCTION AND SCOPE
Geriatric Suicide

Suicide, the deliberate act of causing death by self-injurious behavior, is more common in geriatric patients than in young people.[1] In the United States, each year more than 7000 persons aged 60 and older commit suicide.[2] Older adults also have high rates of suicide worldwide.[3] A 2010 study revealed that, in the elderly population, 1 intentional death by suicide occurs every 1.5 hours.[1] Suicide ranks ninth among causes of death in the United States, ahead of sepsis, liver disease, and hypertension.[4] The National Hospital Ambulatory Medical Care Survey estimates that, in

Disclosure Statement: The authors have nothing to disclose.
[a] Division of Trauma and Surgical Critical Care, Texas Tech University Health Sciences Center, 3601 4th Street MS 8312, Lubbock, TX 79430, USA; [b] Division of Acute Care Surgery, Loma Linda University Medical Center, 11175 Campus Street, CP 21109, Loma Linda, CA 92350, USA
* Corresponding author.
E-mail address: kmukherjee@llu.edu

Clin Geriatr Med 35 (2019) 133–145
https://doi.org/10.1016/j.cger.2018.08.012
0749-0690/19/© 2018 Elsevier Inc. All rights reserved.

2005, there were 575,000 visits to US hospital emergency departments for self-inflicted injuries.[5] From 1999 through 2014, suicide rates have increased by 25%.[6]

Unfortunately, geriatric patients commit suicide more often than their younger counterparts. Although there may be as many as 200 attempted suicides for each suicidal death in adolescents and young adults, the elderly are much more deliberate in their efforts. In contrast, for every 2 to 4 elderly who attempt suicide, 1 is successful.[7] This startling statistic may be due to the greater isolation associated with old age, such that no one is around to detect or rescue the individual at risk. The degree of "successful suicide" among the elderly might also be due to frailty, in which they are less able to tolerate the stress of violent self-harm injuries.[8] Geriatric patients are also more likely to use more lethal means of attempting suicide than younger persons. A 2010 study revealed that younger people commit suicide by firearm 46.7% of the time, whereas 71.4% of geriatric suicides involved the use of a firearm.[7] In addition, geriatric patients have alterations in their anatomy, physiology, and response to trauma and critical illness that decrease their likelihood of recovery or survival from a suicide attempt.[9] Our ability to predict the outcome of geriatric trauma patients, including those with attempted self-harm, is limited owing to maladaptation of traditional mortality scoring systems for the elderly, and this factor in turn impairs our ability as providers to care for them in their moment of crisis.[10,11]

Importance of Prevention

All these factors have underscored the importance of suicide prevention, as well as identification of high-risk individuals who can be targeted for intervention before they make an attempt on their life. This loss of life has an emotional toll on surviving family and friends. Suicide is a preventable public health issue and may be addressed with interventions that improve the detection of patients with suicidal ideation, promote prevention, provide resilience training, and enlist community-based efforts. Suicidal behavior is complex and numerous etiologies must be considered when discussing suicidal behavior and prevention.

IDENTIFICATION OF HIGH-RISK PATIENTS
Difficulties with Identification

The identification of high-risk patients is the first step in suicide prevention. However, such identification is not straightforward. Frequently, it involves screening the elderly patient in a clinic visit or nursing home encounter before the patient's suicidal ideation is promulgated into a suicide attempt or death. Primary care providers (PCPs) and nursing homes are the gatekeepers for suicide prevention and must inquire about mental illness and suicidal ideation.[12] This inquiry is more subtle and complex than it would otherwise seem, because elderly patients may report physical symptoms rather than classical depressive symptoms, making identification of high-risk patients difficult.[13] Thus, trained providers who are aware of such challenges may improve the detection of those at risk for suicide in both nursing homes and traditional clinic settings, where the implementation of suicide prevention methods are most useful.[14]

The Beck Hopelessness Scale and Geriatric Depression Scale can be used for assessment purposes. The Beck scale offers 20 relatively straightforward true/false questions. Although suicide is never directly referenced, the scale assesses how the subject views the future—darkly or with hope, pleasant or unpleasant. The Geriatric Depression Scale attempts to detect precursors for suicide by assessing for hopelessness with questions such as, "Do you see any future for yourself?" or "Do you have any hope?" It then transitions to assessment of the level of passive desire to be dead, asking "Do you ever wish you could just go to sleep and not wake up?" and similar questions. Finally, it offers traditional questions assessing for the presence, duration, frequency, and severity of suicidal ideation. Although other scales exist, these 2 instruments have been in use for the greatest duration (since 1974 in the case of the Beck scale) and have also been validated in multiple studies.[15,16] There is a strong correlation between depressive symptoms and suicide as measured by the Geriatric Depression Scale.[17]

By making these assessment tools relatively straightforward and available to the screening practitioner, it is hoped that patients who display the early signs of suicidality can be identified and helped before proceeding with an attempted suicide. It is also notable that these tests do not require a great deal of training to administer or interpret and, therefore, could be easily administered by an advanced practice clinician.

High-Risk Subpopulations

Not all elderly persons have the same likelihood of being successfully identified with random screening interventions. There are subpopulations within the elderly in which suicide risk is more difficult to assess. An example is the elderly patient with preexisting dementia. According to Alphs and colleagues,[18] our current terminology, practice patterns, and assessment tools may not be sufficient to adequately assess suicide risk in dementia patients, which is 8 times more common than in the general elderly population. Existing suicide risk assessments, including the Beck scale and the Geriatric Depression Scale, have either inadequate assessment of the degree of suicidal ideation, poor risk stratification, low correlation with suicide behavior, or a lack of validation in those with dementia. Alphs and his co-authors,[18] although representing a task force, recommended additional research in this high-risk subpopulation to ensure that patients with suicidality are not overlooked.

Screening for Suicide: Subject to Interpretation

In addition to concerns regarding the efficacy of the diagnostic tools available to physicians and other professionals involved in risk screening for suicide, there are also concerns about how the results of these screening tests are interpreted. In a survey of academic PCPs, 94% were able to detect suicidal ideation in vignettes simulating a young patient and an old patient. However, providers were significantly less likely ($P < .001$) to initiate treatment for the older patient. Reasons for this possible provider bias included normalization of the suicidal statements made by the older patient and belief that treatment for the elderly would be less effective. This finding validates other studies in which improved primary care depression diagnosis education did not result in increased referral to mental health professionals. The problem may be a lack of faith in those very same mental health professionals and their ability to treat the elderly.[19] Future educational efforts might focus on outcomes, rather than the indications, for depression treatment in the elderly.

RISK FACTORS AND PREVENTION
Mental Illness

Depression and social isolation are consistent independent risk factors for suicidal behavior.[20] One key risk factor is unrecognized, and therefore untreated, depression.[7] The family members and friends of those at risk have been shown to accurately recognize this risk. Studies emphasize that when an elderly patient's social support proxy believes the patient is at high risk for depression or suicidal ideation, there is a strong correlation with actual depression and real suicidal ideation.[21] Therefore, clinicians should question an elderly patient's proxy regarding signs and symptoms of depression or suicidal ideation in the patient and act urgently to prevent self-harm in those who are deemed to be at high risk.[21]

Suicidal ideation is another key risk factor for suicide in the elderly, and self-reported suicidal ideation has been associated with death within 1 year.[22] Unfortunately, the elderly are less likely to report their suicidal thoughts.[23] Of older patients who successfully commit suicide, 50% to 75% have seen their PCP within 1 month of the act.[1] Therefore, PCPs are crucial in the identification, assessment, and management of elderly patients at risk for suicide. PCPs might identify increasing functional impairments, severe chronic pain, alcohol abuse and dependence, and depression and other mood disorders. Aggressive treatment plans, intervention with social workers, or assertion of influence can decrease the likely of the patient proceeding with self-harm. Although male sex is a major risk for suicide, with men committing suicide 6 times more often than women, there are numerous other important risk factors related to death by self-directed violence.[2] Additional risk factors for suicide in the elderly include moderate to severe depression, suicidal ideation, thwarted belongingness (feeling disconnected from meaningful social relationships), perceived burdensomeness (feeling a burden or liability to others), psychiatric illness, medical illness, life stressors, and functional impairment (disability).[1,7]

Mental illness patterns also change with age. A study of veterans with schizophrenia revealed that the prevalence of hallucinations was less in the elderly subset of patients, although it was not studied how this change in disease presentation affected suicidality directly.[24] Suicide has a high prevalence in elderly patients with schizophrenia, especially those with a dual diagnosis of schizophrenia and a mood disorder and those who have previous suicide attempts.[25]

In a unique study, elderly survivors of attempted suicide were found to have a 7-fold increased risk of dementia later in life, independent of depression and lack of dementia history.[26] These factors indicate that there remains much to learn about disease effects and their treatments on the elderly. An improved understanding of the presentation and pattern of psychiatric diseases that occur in the elderly may help providers to more easily detect those at risk of suicidal behavior, and thus save lives.

Treatments for mental illness, including depression, carry a risk. A large population-based study of insurance and billing records from Canada's centralized health care system indicated that elderly patients undergoing depression treatment with selective serotonin reuptake inhibitors were at a 5-fold increased suicide risk during the first month of therapy compared with patients treated with other antidepressants.[27] A complex, propensity score-based matching system compared more than 20 other variables in this analysis to isolate the effect of depression medical treatment. Thus, the signs, symptoms, effects, and treatments of mental illness have a complex interplay with suicidal behavior and even future mental illness, emphasizing that those patients identified on screening to be at risk for suicidal behavior should be referred promptly to mental health professionals.

Firearms

Depressive symptoms in the setting of firearm access can be a lethal combination. Access to firearms is associated with increased risk for suicide at all ages.[28,29] PCPs are in a unique position to inquire about firearm possession and firearm safety. Firearm safety counseling could potentially be provided both inside and outside PCP offices. The "5 Ls" framework can be used to identify older adults potentially at risk for firearm injury.[29] The 5 Ls framework addresses firearm storage (locked and loaded); presence of children in the home (little children), suicidal thoughts and prior attempts (feeling low), and prior firearm safety training (learned operator).

It is worth noting that numerous physician organizations have issued statements within the past 5 years concerning firearm violence. The Western Trauma Association recently advocated the reinstitution of a ban on assault weapons, high-capacity magazines, and bump stocks that allow semiautomatic weapons to be easily used in a de facto automatic mode.[30] The American College of Surgeons, in addition to supporting a ban on assault weapons and high-capacity magazines, has advocated more stringent mandatory background checks at gun shows and auctions, more aggressive referral practices for patients identified at screening to have mental health issues, education efforts aimed at safe gun storage and nonviolent conflict resolution, and evidence-based research on firearm injury, including a nationwide firearm injury database (**Fig. 1**).[31] The American Association for the Surgery of Trauma has recommended ending congressional restrictions to the funding of firearm injury research and augmenting the National Violent Death Reporting System, as well as widespread adoption of the Stop the Bleed campaign inaugurated at the Hartford consensus.[32]

Inspired by numerous recent incidents of mass shootings at schools and other public venues, some of these recommendations may also promote suicide prevention. For instance, background checks might identify individuals with a past history of violence and thus result in earlier and more frequent referrals to mental health professionals. Finally, the phenomenon of murder–suicide is also relevant. In a large literature review, the incidence of murder–suicides in those greater than 55 years of age was twice that

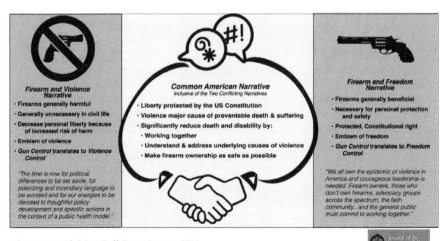

Fig. 1. The American College of Surgeons firearms statement in cartoon format illustrates the common narratives on both sides of the firearms intervention debate and emphasizes the need for broadly supported, common sense interventions that could save lives. (*From* Journal of the American College of Surgeons. August JACS: effective violence-related injury prevention requires engagement, responsibility, and partnership across disciplines, geographic regions, and philosophic differences. Available at: https://twitter.com/jamcollsurg/status/1023342514928078849. Accessed August 6, 2018; with permission.)

in younger patients, and between 85.8% and 100.0% of murder–suicides reported in the medical literature used firearms.[33,34] Like other firearm-related suicides, there is significant male predominance.[35] Measures that decrease the lethality of firearms, such as the reinstitution of an assault weapons ban, might decrease the effectiveness of some murder–suicides as well. Therefore, a more aggressive approach to violence prevention in our society might provide numerous benefits and help to avoid tragic loss of life.

Physical Illness

In addition to mental illness, physical illnesses such as malignancy, male genital disorders, chronic obstructive pulmonary disease, neurologic disorders, arthritis, and functional impairments may all escalate the feeling of social isolation and increase suicide risk.[36,37] These observations exist in studies and systematic reviews of more than 60 studies. Similarly, 23% of Medicare patients undergoing home health follow-up visits claimed passive or active suicidal ideation in a randomized study of 306 patients; these patients typically have other medical conditions requiring prolonged home nursing care.[38] Simply having a chronic disease may not be the only factor involved. Notably, restrictions in physical activity owing to chronic disease (and not necessarily the chronic disease itself) were associated with a doubling of the odds ratio of suicidal ideation in a study of elderly Korean patients.[39]

Socioeconomic Factors

Socioeconomic factors are also relevant in the assessment of suicide risk. Family discord is a major risk factor for suicide among elderly men and women.[40,41] Job loss and financial instability were also identified as a significant risk factors in a European study. There was also a geographic influence exhibited as individuals from the Estonian arm of the study were at higher risk than in the German arm.[42] The long-lasting psychosocial effects of child abuse and neglect, sexual violence, depression, and disrupted social networks also contribute to suicidal behavior.[43,44]

Cognitive and Executive Dysfunction

Even with the identification of these risk factors, impulsive suicide attempts have been reported in older people with central nervous system frontal executive dysfunction secondary to poor cognitive function and poor executive performance.[45] These suicide attempts could not be attributed to the presence of dementia, depression, substance abuse, medication exposure, or other brain disorders. In older veterans, poor cognitive functioning and greater mental distress, as determined by clinical testing and poorer self-perception of physical health, were strongly associated with both passive and active suicidal ideation ($P < .001$) in a study of more than 15,000 outpatients.[46] Older adults with cognitive impairments and later-life depression may benefit from problem solving therapy. Gustavson and colleagues[47] showed that the problem solving therapy group had a significant decrease in suicide ideation both during treatment and at 24 weeks after treatment.

Protective Factors

It is also noteworthy that societal or cultural concerns may serve as protective factors against suicide. Elderly Taiwanese outpatients in unhappy situations were interviewed in a qualitative fashion to explore reasons why individuals experiencing stressors might find motivation to live rather than ending their life.[48] Six major themes were identified as protective factors: being satisfied with one's life, understanding that suicide cannot resolve problems, fear of humiliating one's children, strong religious beliefs, not having previously thought about suicide, and living in harmony with nature. These findings may reflect the unique aspects of community interaction in a different cultural setting. Thus, there may be corresponding features in other cultures or social sub-groups that have a similar effect.

MULTIDISCIPLINARY INTERVENTIONS
Connections to the Community

Social connectedness is crucial for decreasing suicide risk. Community engagement enhances physical health, reduces stress, and decreases depressive symptoms.[49] Connectivity is a primary component of suicide prevention programs for adults who present after nonfatal suicidal behaviors.[50] Motto and Bostrom[50] showed that patients who remained in the ongoing contact group had reduced rates of suicide for at least 2 years. A study of elderly Koreans indicated that those who failed to obtain standard preventive care and follow-up for their chronic medical conditions had a greater risk of suicide. As a result, targeted interventions were placed in the community to ensure easier access for the patients in question.[51]

In Japan, a comprehensive suicide prevention initiative promotes connection to others in the community.[52] This program includes educational health workshops, a commitment among elderly neighbors to be aware of their own and others suicide risk, and depression screening and treatment. Over the decade after implementation, the town of Jojobi noted a 73% (95% confidence interval, 6%–92%) relative risk reduction in suicide mortality for elderly men and a 76% (95% confidence interval, 41%–90%) for elderly women. Kim and Yang[53] developed a small group, focused suicide prevention program for elders with early stage dementia. This program included family support, regional community support, evaluation and treatment of depression, improvement in perceived health status, and activities of daily living. Sessions were held twice weekly for 5 weeks and the treatment group showed significant increases in their perceived health status and social support, coupled with significant decreases in depression and suicidal ideation. Helpline services with trained staff providing brief telephonic counseling also allow for identification of individuals at high risk for suicide with the opportunity to refer them to further timely interventions.[54]

Insurance: The Mental Health Equalizer

Health insurance policies also vary in their coverage of mental health conditions. When states enacted mental health parity laws that required coverage of mental health conditions on par with coverage of physical ailments, self-reported use of mental health care services significantly increased.[55] A similar response was noted in response to federal parity legislation with relatively few incidents of noncompliance.[56] The Affordable Care Act was likewise seen as potentially revolutionary via its enhancement of mental health coverage, although numerous problems remain with lack of coverage, implementation, and enforcement.[57] Ensuring adequate access to affordable, high-quality mental health care will be crucial to any population-based effort to decrease the burden of suicide in our society.

Multidisciplinary Protocols for Intervention

Direct intervention by social workers, nurses, and psychologists has been shown to decrease suicidal ideation and lower rates of major depression. Interventions included suicide assessments and treatment of depression with pharmacotherapy or psycho-therapy.[58] Frequently, a multidisciplinary, community-based approach is necessary to achieve meaningful change.[49]

The Department of Psychiatry at Henry Ford Health System introduced an innovative and comprehensive method of identifying high-risk patients, broad implementation of suicide prevention protocols across inpatient and outpatient facilities, treatment with pharmacotherapy, psychotherapy, a website to connect patients directly with the resources and support, and a partnership with the insurance division of the health system.[59] The suicide rate decreased by 75% during this time period. This type of coordinated care has been applied in other settings as well; patients in the arm of the PROSPECT randomized clinical trial who received coordinated care from a panel of case managers offering protocol-based recommendations to treating physicians were much more likely to receive antidepressants or psychotherapy and, likely because of this increased use of medical treatment, experienced a more than 2-fold decrease in suicidal ideation as compared with patients who received usual care.[58]

Other brief interventions are also effective in decreasing suicide attempts. Patients who have previously attempted suicide are identified and a brief intervention is performed providing psychosocial counseling and supportive ongoing contact.[60] This includes a 1-hour discharge information session addressing suicidal ideation and attempts, distress, risk and protective factors, alternatives to self-harm, and referral options as well as follow-up contact. Fleischmann and colleagues[60] showed a decrease in suicide deaths up to 18 months after discharge from the emergency department with this method. Social inequalities are also linked with major depression and suicide, reemphasizing the need for access to medical care to identify and treat mental health conditions.[61]

Options to Manage Resources

Multidisciplinary interventions of the type discussed elsewhere in this article are highly resource intensive. Unfortunately, there is a significant shortage of mental health providers, and this shortage is most keenly felt in low-income urban and rural communities.[62] Telemedicine, however, may help to bridge this gap, allowing a limited number of providers to access patients across a broader geographic area, particularly if they are not able to attend standard clinic visits.[63] A telephone-based keypad device that allowed participants to answer questions about their health on a daily basis had relatively high adherence and resulted in an improvement in suicidal ideation scores.[64] A telehealth service that provided phone calls to 18,641 patients twice a week as well as 24-hour emergency assistance if needed over a 10-year period resulted in significantly fewer suicide deaths (28.8% standardized mortality ratio for those using the service; $P < .001$).[65]

Additionally, advance practice clinicians may be an option to serve the gatekeeper role described elsewhere in this article. Many advance practice nurses have taken up primary care roles in locations as disparate as clinics, universities, and pharmacies. Geriatric patients will only infrequently seek help directly from mental health professionals, so advance practice clinicians have a crucial role to play in screening for suicidal ideation and referring potentially suicidal patients to specialists in the field.[66] Interestingly, physicians and nurse practitioners also complement each other in the treatment of potentially suicidal elderly patients. Physicians tend to rely on psychotropic medications to treat depression and to refer patients requiring specialist care to their psychiatry colleagues. Nurse practitioners used a more varied approach; although they were less likely to refer to psychiatrists and hospitals and less likely to refer depressed patients to providers performing electroconvulsive therapy, they relied more on interdisciplinary collaboration, including crisis management teams and social workers.[67]

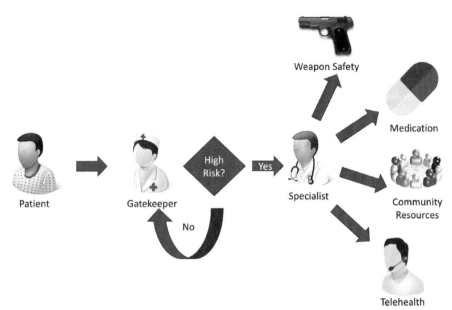

Fig. 2. In this cartoon, a patient sees his or her primary care provider (PCP), who may be a physician or physician extender. This provider screens the patient for potential suicide risk. Low-risk patients are followed up by the PCP. High-risk patients are referred promptly to a mental health professional, who initiates a multidisciplinary community-based set of interventions. These interventions may include medications, options to increase connectedness in the community, firearms safety interventions, and follow-up with telehealth interventions to extend the reach of the mental health professional.

SUMMARY

With the number of elderly patients projected to increase into the foreseeable future, the importance of suicide risk assessment and prevention in this population is paramount. The authors envision an organized paradigm (**Fig. 2**) in which a patient approaches a PCP who may be a physician or advance practice clinician. Screening questions yield a determination of which patients are high risk and ought to be referred to a specialist. The specialist, in turn, initiates a multidisciplinary and collaborative care pathway involving medical therapy, community resources, and discussions regarding safety in the setting of highly lethal and available weapons. Telehealth is a possible option for follow-up of these patients with high availability and low cost. However, such a pathway requires a societal investment in the mental health and well-being of our elderly; legislative and insurance-based solutions to increase access may yield substantial benefits and ultimately save lives.

REFERENCES

1. Carlson WL, Ong TD. Suicide in later life: failed treatment or rational choice? Clin Geriatr Med 2014;30(3):553–76.
2. Karch D. Sex differences in suicide incident characteristics and circumstances among older adults: surveillance data from the national violent death reporting system—17 U.S. States, 2007–2009. Int J Environ Res Public Health 2011;8(8): 3479–95.

3. Heisel MJ, Conwell Y, Pisani AR, et al. Concordance of self- and proxy-reported suicide ideation in depressed adults 50 years of age or older. Can J Psychiatry 2011;56(4):219–26.
4. National Center for Health Statistics. 10 leading causes of injury deaths by age group highlighting unintentional injury deaths. Available at: https://www.cdc.gov/nchs/fastats. Accessed June 30, 2018.
5. National Center for Health Statistics. Suicide and self-inflicted injury. Available at: https://www.cdc.gov/nchs/fastats/suicide. Accessed June 30, 2018.
6. Curtin S, Warner M, Hedegaard H. Increase in suicide in the United States, 1999-2014. NCHS Data Brief 2016;(241):1–8. Available at: https://www.cdc.gov/nchs/fastats.
7. Conwell Y. Suicide later in life. Am J Prev Med 2014;47(Supplement):S244–50.
8. Maxwell CA, Mion LC, Mukherjee K, et al. Preinjury physical frailty and cognitive impairment among geriatric trauma patients determine postinjury functional recovery and survival. J Trauma Acute Care Surg 2016;80(2):195–203.
9. Brooks SE, Peetz AB. Evidence-based care of geriatric trauma patients. Surg Clin North Am 2017;97(5):1157–74.
10. Brooks SE, Mukherjee K, Gunter OL, et al. Do models incorporating comorbidities outperform those incorporating vital signs and injury pattern for predicting mortality in geriatric trauma? J Am Coll Surg 2014;219(5):1020–7.
11. Madni TD, Ekeh AP, Brakenridge SC, et al. A comparison of prognosis calculators for geriatric trauma: a prognostic assessment of life and limitations after trauma in the elderly consortium study. J Trauma Acute Care Surg 2017;83(1):90–6.
12. Lapierre S, Erlangsen A, Wærn M, et al. A systematic review of elderly suicide prevention programs. Crisis 2011;32(2):88–98.
13. Grossberg GT, Beck D, Zaidi SNY. Rapid depression assessment in geriatric patients. Clin Geriatr Med 2017;33(3):383–91.
14. Chauliac N, Brochard N, Payet C, et al. How does gatekeeper training improve suicide prevention for elderly people in nursing homes? A controlled study in 24 centres. Eur Psychiatry 2016;37:56–62.
15. Pérez Rodríguez S, Marco Salvador JH, García-Alandete J. The role of hopelessness and meaning in life in a clinical sample with non-suicidal self-injury and suicide attempts. Psicothema 2017;29(3):323–8.
16. Beck AT, Weissman A, Lester D, et al. The measurement of pessimism: the hopelessness scale. J Consult Clin Psychol 1974;42(6):861–5.
17. Yi S-W. Depressive symptoms on the geriatric depression scale and suicide deaths in older middle-aged men: a prospective cohort study. J Prev Med Public Health 2016;49(3):176–82.
18. Alphs L, Brashear HR, Chappell P, et al. Considerations for the assessment of suicidal ideation and behavior in older adults with cognitive decline and dementia. Alzheimers Dement (N Y) 2016;2(1):48–59.
19. Uncapher H, Areán PA. Physicians are less willing to treat suicidal ideation in older patients. J Am Geriatr Soc 2000;48(2):188–92.
20. Conwell Y, Duberstein PR, Caine ED. Risk factors for suicide in later life. Biol Psychiatry 2002;52(3):193–204.
21. Reske-Nielsen C, Medzon R. Geriatric trauma. Emerg Med Clin North Am 2016;34(3):483–500.
22. Wærn M, Beskow J, Runeson B, et al. Suicidal feelings in the last year of life in elderly people who commit suicide. Lancet 1999;354(9182):917–8.

23. Shah R, Franks P, Jerant A, et al. The effect of targeted and tailored patient depression engagement interventions on patient–physician discussion of suicidal thoughts: a randomized control trial. J Gen Intern Med 2014;29(8):1148–54.
24. Fraser C. Risk factors for suicide in older inpatient veterans with schizophrenia. Community Ment Health J 2018. https://doi.org/10.1007/s10597-018-0267-3.
25. Kiosses DN, Szanto K, Alexopoulos GS. Suicide in older adults: the role of emotions and cognition. Curr Psychiatry Rep 2014;16(11):495.
26. Tu Y-A, Chen M-H, Tsai C-F, et al. Geriatric suicide attempt and risk of subsequent dementia: a nationwide longitudinal follow-up study in Taiwan. Am J Geriatr Psychiatry 2016;24(12):1211–8.
27. Juurlink DN, Mamdani MM, Kopp A, et al. The risk of suicide with selective serotonin reuptake inhibitors in the elderly. Am J Psychiatry 2006;163(5):813–21.
28. Anestis MD, Anestis JC. Suicide rates and state laws regulating access and exposure to handguns. Am J Public Health 2015;105(10):2049–58.
29. Lum HD, Flaten HK, Betz ME. Research article gun access and safety practices among older adults. Curr Gerontol Geriatr Res 2016;1–5. https://doi.org/10.1155/2016/2980416.
30. Western Trauma Association. Western trauma association resolution regarding assault weapons; 2018. Available at: http://www.westerntrauma.org/documents/WTAAssaultWeaponsResolution.pdf. Accessed September 25, 2018.
31. American College of Surgeons. Statement on firearm injuries. Bull Am Coll Surg 2013;98(3):65.
32. Streib E, Blake D, Christmas AB, et al. American association for the Surgery of trauma statement on firearm injuries. J Trauma Acute Care Surg 2016;80(6):849–51.
33. Eliason S. Murder-suicide: a review of the recent literature. J Am Acad Psychiatry Law 2009;37(3):371–6.
34. De Koning E, Piette MH. A retrospective study of murder–suicide at the Forensic Institute of Ghent University, Belgium: 1935–2010. Med Sci Law 2013;54(2):88–98.
35. Oliffe JL, Han CSE, Drummond M, et al. Men, masculinities, and murder-suicide. Am J Mens Health 2015;9(6):473–85.
36. Conwell Y, Duberstein PR, Hirsch JK, et al. Health status and suicide in the second half of life. Int J Geriatr Psychiatry 2010;25(4):371–9.
37. Fässberg MM, Cheung G, Canetto SS, et al. A systematic review of physical illness, functional disability, and suicidal behaviour among older adults. Aging Ment Health 2015;20(2):166–94.
38. Lohman MC, Raue PJ, Greenberg RL, et al. Reducing suicidal ideation in home health care: results from the CAREPATH depression care management trial. Int J Geriatr Psychiatry 2015;31(7):708–15.
39. Jang SY, Choi B, Ju E-Y, et al. Association between restriction of activity related to chronic diseases and suicidal ideation in older adults in Korea. Geriatr Gerontol Int 2014;14(4):983–8.
40. Rubenowitz E, Waern M, Wilhelmson K, et al. Life events and psychosocial factors in elderly suicides–a case control study. Psychol Med 2001;31(7):1193–202.
41. Conejero I, Olié E, Courtet P, et al. Suicide in older adults: current perspectives. Clin Interv Aging 2018;13:691–9.
42. Kõlves K, Värnik A, Schneider B, et al. Recent life events and suicide: a case-control study in Tallinn and Frankfurt. Soc Sci Med 2006;62(11):2887–96.
43. Chapman DP, Whitfield CL, Felitti VJ, et al. Adverse childhood experiences and the risk of depressive disorders in adulthood. J Affect Disord 2004;82(2):217–25.

44. Dube SR, Anda RF, Felitti VJ, et al. Childhood abuse, household dysfunction, and the risk of attempted suicide throughout the life span: findings from the adverse childhood experiences study. JAMA 2001;286(24):3089–96.

45. Dombrovski AY, Butters MA, Reynolds CF III, et al. Cognitive performance in suicidal depressed elderly: preliminary report. Am J Geriatr Psychiatry 2008;16(2):109–15.

46. Ayalon L, Mackin S, Arean PA, et al. The role of cognitive functioning and distress in suicidal ideation in older adults. J Am Geriatr Soc 2007;55(7):1090–4.

47. Gustavson KA, Alexopoulos GS, Niu GC, et al. Problem-solving therapy reduces suicidal ideation in depressed older adults with executive dysfunction. Am J Geriatr Psychiatry 2016;24(1):11–7.

48. Chen Y-J, Tsai Y-F, Lee S-H, et al. Protective factors against suicide among young-old Chinese outpatients. BMC Public Health 2014;14:372.

49. Centers for Disease Control. Principles of community engagement. Atlanta (GA): Centers for Disease Control; 2011. Available at: https://www.atsdr.cdc.gov/communityengagement/pdf/PCE_Report_FINAL.pdf. Accessed September 25, 2018.

50. Motto JA, Bostrom AG. A randomized controlled trial of postcrisis suicide prevention. Psychiatr Serv 2001;52(6):828–33.

51. Park S-M, Moon S-S. Elderly Koreans who consider suicide_ Role of healthcare use and financial status. Psychiatry Res 2016;244(C):345–50.

52. Oyama H, Koida J, Sakashita T, et al. Community-based prevention for suicide in elderly by depression screening and follow-up. Community Ment Health J 2004;40(3):249–63.

53. Kim J-P, Yang J. Effectiveness of a community-based program for suicide prevention among elders with early-stage dementia: a controlled observational study. Geriatr Nurs 2017;38(2):97–105.

54. Chan C-H, Wong H-K, Yip PS-F. Exploring the use of telephone helpline pertaining to older adult suicide prevention_ A Hong Kong experience. J Affect Disord 2018;236:75–9.

55. Harris KM, Carpenter C, Bao Y. The effects of state parity laws on the use of mental health care. Med Care 2006;44(6):499–505.

56. Hodgkin D, Horgan CM, Stewart MT, et al. Federal parity and access to behavioral health care in private health plans. Psychiatr Serv 2018;69(4):396–402.

57. Rochefort DA. The affordable care act and the faltering revolution in behavioral health care. Int J Health Serv 2018;48(2):223–46.

58. Alexopoulos GS, Reynolds CF, Bruce ML, et al. Reducing suicidal ideation and depression in older primary care patients: 24-month outcomes of the PROSPECT study. Am J Psychiatry 2009;166(8):882–90.

59. Coffey CE. Pursuing perfect depression care. Psychiatr Serv 2006;57(10):1524–6.

60. Fleischmann A, Bertolote JM, Wasserman D, et al. Effectiveness of brief intervention and contact for suicide attempters: a randomized controlled trial in five countries. Bull World Health Organ 2008;86(9):703–9.

61. Gilman SE, Bruce ML, Have TT, et al. Social inequalities in depression and suicidal ideation among older primary care patients. Soc Psychiatry Psychiatr Epidemiol 2012;48(1):59–69.

62. Health resources and services administration. Shortage areas. Available at: https://datawarehouse.hrsa.gov/topics/shortageareas.aspx. Accessed July 12, 2018.

63. Hailey D, Roine R, Ohinmaa A. The effectiveness of telemental health applications: a review. Can J Psychiatry 2008;53(11):769–78.
64. Kasckow J, Zickmund S, Gurklis J, et al. Using telehealth to augment an intensive case monitoring program in veterans with schizophrenia and suicidal ideation: a pilot trial. Psychiatry Res 2016;239:111–6.
65. De Leo D, Buono Dello M, Dwyer J. Suicide among the elderly: the long-term impact of a telephone support and assessment intervention in northern Italy. Br J Psychiatry 2002;181:226–9.
66. Boxwell AO. Geriatric suicide: the preventable death. Nurse Pract 1988;13(6): 10–1, 15, 18–9.
67. Adamek ME, Kaplan MS. Caring for depressed and suicidal older patients: a survey of physicians and nurse practitioners. Int J Psychiatry Med 2000;30(2): 111–25.